M000271851

IT STARTS
WITH THE EGG
Fertility Cookbook

100 Mediterranean-Inspired Recipes

IT STARTS
WITH THE EGG
Fertility Cookbook

REBECCA FETT

FRANKLIN
FOX

It Starts with the Egg Fertility Cookbook
Copyright © 2020, Rebecca Fett
First Edition.
www.itstartswiththeegg.com

Published in the United States by Franklin Fox.

All rights reserved. No part of this publication may be reproduced in any form by any means without the express permission of the publisher.

This book is intended to provide helpful and informative material. It is not intended to provide medical advice and cannot replace the advice of a nutritionist or medical professional. The author and publisher specifically disclaim all responsibility for any liability, loss, or risk, personal or otherwise, which is incurred as a consequence of the use and application of any of the contents of this book.

ISBN-13 (print): 978-0-9996761-6-5
ISBN-10 (ebook): 978-0-9996761-7-2

Contents

Introduction

DIET CAN HAVE a profound effect on fertility, impacting both the time it takes to conceive naturally and the odds of success in IVF. This is in part due to the important role of nutrients, such as folate, that are needed for proper egg and embryo development. But choosing the right foods can also help balance hormones, reduce inflammation, and support cellular energy production.

This sounds like a lot to ask from diet alone, but there is clear scientific evidence showing that diet truly is one of the most powerful tools we have when it comes to improving fertility. I have been closely following the scientific studies in this area for many years now, after first delving into the research in order to address my own infertility diagnosis.

Like so many other young women, I initially took my fertility for granted. In my late twenties, when my husband and I were ready to start a family, we had no choice but to pursue gestational surrogacy, since I had health problems that would have made pregnancy quite dangerous. Once we found our surrogate, I assumed the rest of the process would be easy. We simply had to go through IVF to produce embryos to transfer to our surrogate. Since I was young and had no known fertility issues, there was every reason to expect success on the first try. Yet I was in for an unpleasant surprise.

Even though I was just 27, I was diagnosed with diminished ovarian reserve and told that our chances of conceiving through IVF were depressingly low.

Readers of my book *It Starts with the Egg* will know what happened next: I put my training in molecular biology and biochemistry to work and dove into all the latest scientific research on what can be done to improve egg quality and fertility.

I found a vast universe of information on how diet, supplements, and common environmental toxins can impact fertility—information that was not widely known at the time. I put all this information into practice with a regime of new supplements and lifestyle changes. After just a few months, I saw a dramatic turnaround. Ultrasounds and lab tests showed that my fertility was no longer on par with someone in their forties but more in line with my actual age of 27. Our subsequent IVF cycle produced 19 good-quality embryos, eventually leading to my two sons.

I wanted to share all the critical information I had uncovered with other women facing similar challenges, which led me to write *It Starts with the Egg*. That book provides detailed guidance on choosing the right supplements for different situations, along with evidence-based advice on diet and how to avoid common toxins.

Although diet is just one component of my approach to restoring egg quality and fertility, it is an important one. In *It Starts with the Egg*, I wrote about the latest scientific research on diet and fertility, such as the positive effects of minimizing refined carbohydrates and shifting toward a Mediterranean diet. But I know that some people want more practical guidance and detailed advice on exactly what to eat—to go beyond the theory and have a specific template to follow.

I also know that many people become stressed and overwhelmed when making major dietary changes, so I wanted to help ease the transition and allow you to shift toward a healthier diet without feeling deprived. The secret to that is having easy-to-follow and delicious recipes, so you can truly enjoy your new diet.

To that end, I created this new book to supplement *It Starts with the Egg*, with over 100 recipes inspired by the Mediterranean diet, along with answers to all your questions about nutrition and fertility. Research shows that food is one of our most powerful tools to address fertility problems; now we just need to put the research into practice. I hope this book will empower you to do just that.

Part 1

Fertility Nutrition Guide

Chapter 1

Fertility Diet Principles

EVEN THOUGH DIET is only one part of the infertility picture, it is uniquely important because it is something we have the power to change. Although the underlying causes of infertility and recurrent miscarriage are typically beyond our control, the simple everyday decisions about the foods we eat can have a surprisingly large impact on how long it takes to conceive.

A wealth of scientific research shows that making a few key changes to your diet can help rebalance hormones, reduce inflammation, and improve egg quality. In short, the right foods can maximize your chance of success regardless of the specific fertility challenge you face. And the best place to start is with a Mediterranean diet.

There is now clear evidence showing that the Mediterranean diet boosts fertility, with a shorter time to pregnancy in couples trying to conceive naturally and higher success rates in IVF.[1] In the IVF context, the more closely couples follow this way of eating, the more likely they are to produce good-quality embryos and the higher the odds of each embryo transfer leading to a successful pregnancy. The difference in IVF success rates between women who have adopted a Mediterranean diet compared to those who have not is quite dramatic, especially for women under 35. In this age group, following a Mediterranean diet is associated with a 2.7 times higher chance of live birth.[2]

The value in switching to a Mediterranean diet is clear, but there are many misconceptions about what this diet actually entails. This chapter aims to fill that gap and translate the research into an easy-to-follow plan of action.

What Exactly Is the Mediterranean Diet?

In the context of medical research, the Mediterranean diet is not what many people expect. Although it has its roots in Italy, France, Spain, and Greece, it is quite different to the modern-day cuisines in this region, which are often known for red wine, bread, cheese, and pasta.

In the research context, the Mediterranean diet refers to the traditional cuisine of communities bordering the Mediterranean Sea, such as the Greek island of Ikaria and Sardinia, in Italy, as it existed 50 to 100 years ago. Researchers were first inspired to investigate the historical way of eating in these regions after noticing the surprising longevity of people living there. Ikaria, for example, is considered a "blue zone"—one of the five places in the world with the highest concentration of people living to 100.

An array of large-scale studies has now found that following the traditional diet patterns from these regions can reduce the risk of diabetes, cancer, heart disease, and many other modern-day diseases.[3] There are two main reasons why the Mediterranean diet has such profound health benefits.

1. It reduces inflammation.
2. It helps control blood sugar levels.

These are the exact same objectives we have in making dietary changes to boost fertility, so it is not surprising that the Mediterranean diet is also incredibly helpful for couples trying to conceive.

But what does the diet actually entail? The most important components of a Mediterranean diet are these: [4]

- vegetables

- legumes

- fish

- olive oil

- nuts

Beyond these core components, traditional Mediterranean diets differ in how much they emphasize other foods, such as fruit, eggs, dairy, poultry, and other meats. Each of these elements will be discussed in detail in the chapters that follow. In general, however, the Mediterranean diet is quite flexible and can be adapted to suit your personal preferences and nutritional needs. It also encompasses cuisines beyond the Mediterranean region; with many Asian recipes fitting a Mediterranean diet by virtue of emphasizing vegetables and seafood.

Rather than providing bright-line rules, the overall goal is to emphasize nutrient-dense whole foods such as vegetables, healthy fats, and lean proteins, while minimizing

- sugar,

- saturated fat, and

- highly processed foods.

Although red wine is typically considered a part of the Mediterranean diet, it is not encouraged for those trying to conceive, because alcohol intake appears to compromise fertility, at least when consumed regularly.[5] The research in this area has produced conflicting results, but on balance it appears that for both men and women, more than a few drinks per week can reduce the odds of successfully conceiving.[6] Consuming four or more drinks per week also significantly increases the risk of miscarriage.[7]

The Connection Between Blood-Sugar and Fertility

As explained in more detail in *It Starts with the Egg*, managing blood sugar levels is one of the most important goals in adopting a fertility-friendly diet. Studies have found that women undergoing IVF who have higher blood sugar levels and a higher intake of sugar and other refined carbohydrates typically end up with fewer eggs retrieved, fewer eggs fertilized, and fewer good-quality embryos.[8] Similarly, men with higher sugar intake have often shown compromised sperm quality.[9]

There are several explanations for this. Part of the problem is that high blood sugar levels trigger surges of insulin, which then disrupts the careful balance of reproductive hormones. This is most evident in women with PCOS, but high insulin levels can contribute to infertility in other women too.

High blood sugar itself can also directly compromise egg quality. That is because it can damage mitochondria—the tiny energy-producing factories inside every cell that are vital to proper egg development.

But addressing this problem does not necessarily require drastically cutting carbohydrates. Instead, the key is choosing the right kinds of carbohydrates and eating well-balanced meals that include protein and healthy fats.

A general goal while trying to conceive is to obtain 40 percent of calories from carbohydrates, and at least 30 percent from protein. This leaves approximately 30 percent of calories from fat. One study found that a small group of women who adopted this ratio, by reducing their normal carbohydrate intake and adding more protein, showed a significant improvement in the number of good-quality embryos and a higher pregnancy rate after IVF.[10]

Yet there is no need to achieve these exact percentages or closely track macronutrients in order to balance blood sugar levels. Rather than focusing on restriction or following rigid rules, a better approach is to emphasize overall diet quality and create balanced, healthy meals.

One way to do so is by using a "balanced plate" as a guide.

To support healthy hormones, a balanced meal should ideally have these components:

- ½ plate non-starchy vegetables

- ¼ plate protein (25 to 30 grams per meal)

- ¼ plate nutrient-dense fruit, legumes, starchy vegetables, or whole grains

- 1 to 2 servings of healthy fat, such as olive oil or avocado

At breakfast, a balanced plate might be simpler, with half protein and half grains or fruit. Examples include Greek yogurt with granola, or eggs with fruit.

In general, creating balanced meals that emphasize vegetables, proteins, healthy fats, and the right types of carbohydrates will not only help you achieve steady blood sugar levels but will also make sure you are getting enough of the nutrients necessary to optimal fertility. By emphasizing the nutrient-dense whole foods that make up the core components of the Mediterranean diet, you will ensure you are getting more of the vitamins, antioxidants, and anti-inflammatory fats that are so beneficial to egg and sperm quality.

The following chapters will delve into each component of the balanced plate, answering the most common questions and providing detailed guidance on exactly what to eat for the best results.

Chapter 2

Non-Starchy Vegetables

Goal: Fill half your plate with colorful, non-starchy vegetables at two meals each day

NUMEROUS STUDIES HAVE found that men and women who eat more vegetables have better IVF outcomes and take less time to conceive if trying naturally. This is likely because vegetables are among the best sources of vitamins, minerals, antioxidants, and fiber, all of which can help improve fertility.

The vegetables with the highest levels of vitamins and antioxidants include

- broccoli,
- cabbage,
- cauliflower,
- kale,
- brussels sprouts,
- asparagus, and
- carrots.

Do I need to buy organic?

Certain pesticides that are used to grow conventional fruit and vegetables are likely endocrine disruptors. This means they could potentially compromise fertility by interfering with the activity of hormones. It is not yet clear that the small amount of pesticide residues on produce would be enough to have an impact on female fertility, but research does suggest a potential problem for sperm quality.

Specifically, researchers have found that men who consume more of the types of fruit and vegetables with the highest levels of pesticides tend to have a lower sperm count and lower percentage of normal sperm morphology.[11] On the other hand, men who eat more low-pesticide fruit and vegetables show better sperm quality.

If budget permits and organic produce is available in your area, it may be worth choosing organic for those vegetables with higher levels of pesticides. These include:

- spinach,
- peppers,
- tomatoes,
- potatoes,
- celery, and
- kale.

There are many other vegetables that typically have low levels of pesticides, in which case buying organic is a low priority. These include:

- avocado,
- onion,
- peas,
- cabbage,
- broccoli,

- asparagus,

- cauliflower, and

- mushrooms.

Is plastic packaging a problem for fruits and vegetables?

The concern over hormone disruptors such as BPA and phthalates in plastics (discussed in detail in *It Starts with the Egg*) leads some people to wonder about the plastic used in food packaging. Fortunately, the research so far suggests that food packaging is not a major source of BPA or phthalates. This is partly because the plastics used are relatively safe, and partly because the chemicals that are present do not seem to transfer in significant amounts to typical foods such as fruit, vegetables, and meats.

The situation is different for foods that are hot or acidic, along with higher-fat liquids, such as milk and oil. All of these items are more likely to absorb chemicals from plastic packaging. For this reason, it is better to purchase milk in cardboard containers and to choose oil, sauces, and condiments in glass bottles whenever possible. As a general rule, however, most chemical contamination of foods comes from contact with plastic during processing, so avoiding highly processed foods in favor of natural, whole ingredients will make the most difference.

Are frozen vegetables as nutritious as fresh?

The vitamin content of frozen vegetables is comparable to fresh and sometimes even higher.[12] The likely explanation for this is that vegetables lose vitamins when stored for long periods at room temperature or in a refrigerator, but less vitamin loss occurs when stored frozen. Very fresh in-season vegetables will likely have the highest vitamin content, but frozen vegetables remain a good choice.

Canned vegetables are the least preferred option because chemicals such as BPA can leach from the can lining. The heat involved in the canning process can also destroy many vitamins, so canned vegetables and fruits are not recommended. The answer is different for canned beans and lentils, however, as discussed later in this chapter.

What are good alternatives to canned tomatoes?

When trying to minimize exposure to BPA and other similar chemicals, canned tomatoes pose a particular concern because the acidity increases leaching from the can lining. The acidity also limits the materials available to manufacturers wishing to avoid BPA, because the safest alternatives are not compatible with highly acidic foods. This means that in the case of tomatoes we have to assume that the can lining probably contains chemicals that are best avoided, even if it says "BPA-free."

The best alternatives to canned tomatoes include using fresh tomatoes, pasta sauce in a glass jar, or tomato salsa in a glass jar. Another acceptable option is to buy tomatoes in a Tetra Pak box. In these boxes, the lining material in contact with the food is typically polyethylene. This is one of the safer types of plastic and an improvement over the chemicals used in the lining of cans, but it is still inferior to glass.

Are nightshades inflammatory?

There is a widespread suspicion that vegetables in the nightshade family, which includes tomatoes, potatoes, and peppers, can worsen inflammation. The autoimmune paleo (AIP) diet therefore eliminates these vegetables, along with nightshade-based spices, such as cayenne and paprika. It is not yet clear whether doing so has any fertility benefits, but it may be worth at least reducing your intake of nightshades if you have an autoimmune or inflammatory condition, such as endometriosis.

The potential link between nightshades and inflammation was first suggested in the 1970s, when a horticulturalist named Norman Childers suspected that his own arthritis was triggered by potatoes, tomatoes, and eggplant.[13] He understood that these were all members of the *Solanaceae* plant family—historically known as nightshades because this family includes the deadly nightshade used by the Romans to poison enemies. There are actually thousands of plants in the nightshade family, many of which are toxic or inedible, such as tobacco.

The edible nightshades include

- tomatoes,

- potatoes (but not sweet potatoes or yams),

- bell peppers/capsicum/sweet peppers,

- chili peppers (and derivative spices such as cayenne, paprika, and chipotle),

- eggplant,

- tomatillos,

- goji berries, and

- ashwaganda (often found in herbal thyroid supplements).

After eliminating all foods from this plant family, Dr. Childers's joint pain rapidly improved. He shared this finding in a book published in the 1970s and in the decades since, thousands of people have reported that they too have reduced the severity of their arthritis by eliminating nightshades. A recent study also found that 52 percent of psoriasis patients reported improvement in their symptoms after eliminating nightshades.[14] Yet there have never been any rigorous scientific studies supporting the link between nightshades and inflammation; all we have to rely on is a plausible biochemical explanation.

This explanation is based on two potentially toxic components found in nightshades: glycoalkaloids and lectins. Both of these groups of chemicals can potentially disrupt the gut barrier and activate the immune system, sparking inflammation. Yet this has only been demonstrated in laboratory and animal studies so far.[15]

There is no definitive answer as to whether nightshades can trigger sufficient inflammation to compromise fertility. Based on what is known so far, it is likely not necessary to strictly eliminate these foods, but it would be reasonable to avoid nightshades if you have an inflammatory condition or want to take a "no-stone-unturned" approach.

Chapter 3

Carbohydrates

Goal: Fill one-quarter of your plate with fruit or high-fiber starches

ALTHOUGH IT IS true that excess sugar and refined carbohydrates can compromise fertility, that does not mean you need to follow a very low-carbohydrate diet while trying to conceive. Instead, a simple and effective strategy is to fill no more than one-quarter of your plate with fruits, beans, lentils, starchy vegetables, or other high-fiber, unprocessed carbohydrates, and the rest of your plate with protein, healthy fats, and non-starchy vegetables. This approach makes it easy to keep the total amount of carbohydrates within a moderate amount, without being overly restrictive.

The research confirms that it only takes a modest reduction in total carbohydrate intake to improve egg quality and fertility. As mentioned earlier, one small study reported higher IVF success rates when women reduced carbohydrate intake to 40 percent of total calories, which translates to approximately 180 to 200 grams of carbohydrates per day.

With this limit, a typical day of meals might look like this:

- Breakfast: 40 g carbohydrates
- Lunch: 60 g carbohydrates
- Snack: 20 g carbohydrates
- Dinner: 80 g carbohydrates

If you emphasize protein and healthy fats at every meal and snack, and keep the carbohydrate portion to approximately one-quarter of your plate at lunch and dinner, it is actually relatively easy to keep total carbohydrate intake within these amounts, as you can see from this example meal plan.

Breakfast

1 cup yogurt and ½ cup granola = 40 g carbohydrates
> OR:

Omelet with 2 eggs and 1 cup mushrooms, plus 1 banana = 30 g carbohydrates

Lunch

Grilled chicken, salad, 1 cup lentils = 50 g carbohydrates

Snack

1 apple, 4 ounces cheese = 20g carbohydrates
> OR:

1 cup strawberries, ½ cup almonds = 26 g carbohydrates

Dinner

Salmon, 1 cup brown rice, 1 cup broccoli = 55 g carbohydrates

Dessert

1 ounce dark chocolate = 13g carbohydrates

Total = 178 g

By relying on protein, vegetables, and healthy fats to make up a significant portion of every meal and snack, you will automatically lower your carbohydrate intake, without needing to keep a count of total grams of carbohydrates and without feeling deprived or hungry.

Combining carbohydrates with protein and vegetables is also a very effective way to minimize the blood sugar impact of the carbohydrates you eat, by slowing down the release of glucose into the bloodstream. Studies have shown that eating carbohydrates 15 minutes after a meal containing protein and vegetables results in a much lower and slower rise in blood glucose levels compared to eating the same amount of carbohydrates on an empty stomach.[16]

The other side to balancing blood sugar levels is choosing the right *types* of carbohydrates, namely those that are broken down slowly. The carbohydrates at the core of the Mediterranean diet—whole grains, fruit, and legumes—are good examples.

Studies show that following a Mediterranean diet lowers the risk of diabetes by at least 60 percent, in large part because it emphasizes these "slow" carbohydrate sources while minimizing refined starches and sugars.[17] Importantly, this ability of the Mediterranean diet to balance insulin levels appears to translate into improved fertility too. Women who rely on high-fiber carbohydrates instead of refined carbohydrates and sugars are significantly more likely to become pregnant over a twelve-month period.[18]

More specifically, the best types of carbohydrate are those with a low "glycemic index," which measures on a scale of 1 to 100 how much impact the food will have on blood glucose levels in a certain amount of time. The lower the number, the better. Studies have found that women who rely more heavily on low-glycemic carbohydrates have a much lower rate of ovulatory infertility.[19]

Typically, the more refined and processed a food is, the higher the glycemic index and the greater the impact on blood sugar and insulin levels. This is because the refining process allows a food to be more rapidly digested, releasing a surge of glucose. On the other hand, high-fiber foods typically have a lower glycemic index because fiber slows the release of glucose.

For this reason, the best choices are typically unprocessed, high-fiber foods, such as

- legumes (beans, lentils, split peas),
- seeds,
- nuts,
- vegetables,
- oats (granola, steel cut oatmeal), and
- fruit.

It is best to limit

- juice,
- soda,
- sugar, and
- foods made from refined white flour (bread, crackers, cakes).

Although it is not necessary to strictly avoid all high-glycemic carbohydrates, you should keep portion size small and make sure to combine these foods with protein and healthy fat. A slice of bread or half a cup of rice is typically not a problem if included as part of a balanced meal, but the same foods could disrupt blood sugar levels when consumed alone or in larger portion sizes.

Starchy vegetables are typically good carbohydrate sources, although some extra attention to portion size is needed in the case of potatoes and sweet potatoes. These particular vegetables are not only very high in carbohydrates, but they also have starches that are quickly broken down, resulting in a sudden spike in blood sugar levels. In some tests, the glycemic index of potato and sweet potato is almost the same as pure glucose. As a result, it is helpful to keep portion size small and rely more heavily on vegetables with a lower glycemic index, such as green peas, pumpkins, carrots, and winter squash.

SMART CARBOHYDRATE SWAPS

Wheat or rice pasta $\longrightarrow$ lentil or chickpea pasta

Bread $\longrightarrow$ paleo or keto bread, seed bread

Crackers $\longrightarrow$ nuts, carrot sticks, flax crackers

Rice $\longrightarrow$ cauliflower rice, lentils

Tortilla $\longrightarrow$ coconut wrap, lettuce wrap

Potatoes $\longrightarrow$ celeriac, turnip, mashed cauliflower, pumpkin

How much fruit can I eat each day?

Although fruit can be high in natural sugars, it is also typically high in fiber, which helps reduce the impact on blood sugar levels. In addition, many fruits are rich in fertility-boosting vitamins and antioxidants, such as vitamin C, folate, and the brightly colored polyphenols found in berries and pomegranate. The benefits of fruit likely outweigh the potential negative impact on blood sugar levels, unless you consume more fruit than your metabolism can handle.

Most people can include two servings of fruit per day without causing blood sugar problems, although you may decide to include more or less, depending on how much you rely on other carbohydrate sources. In one recent study, researchers found that consuming three servings of fruit per day was associated with a shorter time to pregnancy.[20]

To further slow the release of sugars naturally present in fruit, it is helpful to combine fruit with at least some protein, rather than eating it alone on an empty stomach. If you are having fruit as a snack, it is wise to add a small portion of cheese, yogurt, nuts, ham, turkey, or a hardboiled egg, to prevent a sudden spike in blood sugar.

It is also best to choose fresh rather than dried fruit, because the appropriate portion size for dried fruit is quite small, making it all too easy to consume a large amount of sugar. By way of illustration, a small box of raisins has twice as much sugar as one cup of fresh grapes.

Juice is another concentrated source of fruit sugars that should be limited, particularly since it lacks fiber and therefore has more impact on blood sugar. Rather than drinking juice on its own, a good alternative is to mix a small amount of juice with sparkling water. One-quarter cup of pomegranate juice, for example, will have just eight grams of sugar.

Research suggests that the antioxidants found in pomegranates may also have powerful fertility benefits, with studies finding improved sperm quality after men consumed pomegranate extract for three months.[21] There is little direct evidence that pomegranate juice improves fertility for women, but there is reason to be optimistic, given the numerous studies finding that the antioxidants in pomegranates can reduce inflammation and oxidative stress.

Carbohydrate Content of Fruits

1 cup strawberries:	12 g
1 cup grapes:	16 g
1 cup honeydew melon:	16 g
1 peach:	17 g
1 cup blueberries:	21 g
1 cup pineapple:	21 g
1 apple:	25 g
1 banana:	27 g

Does fruit need to be organic?

Although we do not yet know the impact of pesticides on fertility, there are certain fruits that may be worth buying organic when you have the option, out of an abundance of caution. This includes berries and other fruits with a thin, edible peel, which are often contaminated with higher levels of pesticides. By contrast, fruits with a thick peel, such as melons, are usually safe to buy nonorganic, as shown in the list below.

Higher-Pesticide Fruits

- strawberries
- nectarines
- apples
- grapes
- peaches
- cherries
- pears

Lower-Pesticide Fruits

- papaya
- mango
- honeydew
- kiwi
- cantaloupe
- pineapple

For the higher-pesticide fruits, you can also reduce your exposure by removing the peel where possible (such as with apples and pears) or washing with a baking soda solution. To do this, add one teaspoon of baking soda to two cups of water and soak fruit such as berries for 10 to 15 minutes, then rinse and allow to dry on a plate lined with paper towels before storing in the refrigerator.

Are canned beans safe?

Given the concern over BPA and other similar chemicals used in the lining of cans, the general rule is to choose fresh or frozen foods rather than canned, whenever possible. In the case of canned beans, however, the risk/benefit ratio is shifted slightly. That is because beans offer a very nutritious, low-glycemic carbohydrate source, and canned beans are significantly more convenient than cooking dried beans from scratch.

In addition, some manufacturers (such as Eden Organics) have been able to develop safer can linings for beans than for other, more acidic foods. When these factors are considered together, the benefits of using canned beans likely outweighs the downside, especially if you can buy a BPA-free brand. Another good choice is to buy beans in Tetra Paks, such as those by WholeFoods' store brand, 365 Organic.

That said, it is even better to prepare dried beans from scratch, when time allows. Doing so is not only healthier and low cost but also typically produces better results in recipes. The best way to prepare dried beans is to soak them overnight and then cook in a pressure cooker. You can then freeze individual portions for later use.

Are legumes Inflammatory?

Several anti-inflammatory diets, such as the autoimmune paleo (AIP) diet and Whole30, eliminate all legumes on the theory that proteins called lectins can damage the gut and activate the immune system.

Lectins are found in many plants, where they likely serve as a protective mechanism against insects. Although it is possible that lectins in certain foods can be problematic for those with autoimmune or inflammatory conditions, that does not mean it is necessary to eliminate all legumes.

The specific lectins that are most likely to be harmful are those found in pea-nuts, soy, corn, and potatoes. These particular lectins not only survive cooking and digestion but can also cross the gut barrier and activate immune cells, trig-gering inflammation.[22] They also increase intestinal permeability, contributing to so-called "leaky gut."[23]

Yet this problem does not apply to all legumes. Unlike soy and peanut lectins, the lectins found in dried beans can be virtually eliminated by cooking for a sufficient length of time at high heat.[24] Several hours of boiling or 45 minutes of pressure-cooking was found to abolish lectin activity in red kidney beans.[25] It is even easier to deactivate the lectins found in other beans.[26] In 2019, the autoim-mune paleo diet was actually updated to recommend the earlier reintroduction of lentils, peas, and garbanzo beans (chickpeas) on the basis that these lectins are particularly easy to deactivate with heat.

We also know that the fiber and antioxidants present in legumes are very beneficial for the microbiome—the community of beneficial bacteria in our gas-trointestinal system. A vast amount of research has now shown that building a healthy microbiome is one of the best ways to reduce inflammation (discussed in further detail in my autoimmune diet book, *The Keystone Approach*).

Research also shows that diets emphasizing legumes are associated with lower levels of inflammation and reduced symptoms of autoimmune disease, including psoriasis and rheumatoid arthritis.[27] In short, soy and peanuts are likely worth avoiding if you suffer from an autoimmune condition, but other beans and lentils are typically safe to include, especially if soaked and pressure cooked.

As a side note, women with a history of kidney stones, vulvodynia, unexplained joint pain, or chronic bladder conditions may find they feel better avoiding foods that are high in oxalates, which includes certain beans. Oxalates are found in many plant foods, but most people do not absorb them in significant amounts. In those with gut problems, however, oxalates are more readily absorbed, and they can eventually form crystals that trigger bladder, joint, and kidney problems. If you experience these symptoms, it is worth avoiding or limiting kidney, black, cannellini, navy, and pinto beans and instead emphasizing red or brown lentils, split peas, garbanzo beans (chickpeas), and black-eyed peas. Other high-oxalate foods include spinach, chard, beets, nuts, rhubarb, buckwheat, cocoa, and sweet potatoes.

Why is the keto diet often recommended for infertility?

The ketogenic diet is an extremely low-carbohydrate diet that triggers the body to metabolize fat into ketones. A typical keto diet may consist of 75 percent fat, 20 percent protein, and just 5 percent carbohydrates, for a total carbohydrate limit of about 20 to 25 grams per day. This diet, originally developed decades ago as a treatment for epilepsy and diabetes, has gained popularity in recent years as a way to lose weight, reduce inflammation, and control blood sugar levels.

For women with PCOS or diabetes, following a ketogenic diet is often a very effective way to control insulin and glucose levels. This in turn can reduce excess testosterone and restore ovulation.

In 2018, researchers at the Cleveland Clinic investigated the effect of a ketogenic diet in four women with PCOS who had been trying to conceive for an average of three years. Within eight weeks of lowering carbohydrate intake to less than 20 grams per day, the women's previously irregular menstrual cycles normalized. Two of the women went on to become pregnant without any further treatment.[28]

Although this is a very small study, it is consistent with other studies finding that a very low-carbohydrate diet can be beneficial in overweight women with PCOS, resulting in significant weight loss and lower levels of insulin, testosterone, and DHEA.[29] It is not all good news, however, with other studies finding that ketogenic diets can also raise stress hormones and potentially worsen insulin resistance over the long term.[30]

The question for women with PCOS is whether it is necessary to go to the extreme of following a ketogenic diet, or whether a moderately low-carbohydrate diet is enough to reap the benefits of blood sugar and insulin control, which in turn can restore ovulation. We do not yet have a clear answer to this, but research suggests that simply reducing carbohydrates to 40 percent of calories can improve hormone levels in women with PCOS.[31] Adding the other strategies discussed in this chapter, such as carefully choosing carbohydrates that do not cause sudden rises in blood sugar levels and combining carbohydrates with protein and fats, will likely be the best starting point for most women with PCOS.[32]

It is also important to note that the high level of saturated fat that often goes along with a ketogenic diet is likely counterproductive for women with PCOS. As will be discussed in Chapter 5, women with PCOS show a marked increase in inflammation when they consume saturated fat, and this inflammation appears to worsen insulin resistance and other hormonal disruptions.

For those without PCOS, a ketogenic diet is an even riskier approach because it can potentially lower hormones that may already be too low. One such hormone is DHEA, which is an important precursor to reproductive hormones such as testosterone. Although DHEA and testosterone are typically elevated in women with PCOS, and can be decreased with a ketogenic diet, they are more often too low in women with age-related infertility or diminished ovarian reserve.

DHEA is produced by the adrenal glands and it is possible that following a ketogenic diet long term may compromise adrenal function by increasing the demand for cortisol, eventually depleting DHEA levels. Common symptoms of poor adrenal function include extreme fatigue in the afternoon, insomnia, low blood pressure, and craving salt and sugar.

Research also shows that many women following a ketogenic diet develop irregular menstrual cycles or stop having periods altogether.[33] Although we do not yet know why this occurs, it raises a serious red flag and indicates that this diet can profoundly impact reproductive hormones.

Another potential problem with the keto diet is suppressing thyroid hormones. Insulin plays a key role in the conversion of thyroid hormones into their active form. If insulin is too low for too long, as a result of an extremely low-carbohydrate diet, this can cause a drop in active thyroid hormones. We know that a lack of thyroid hormones can be detrimental to fertility and increase the risk of miscarriage.[34]

Not everyone who follows a ketogenic diet will experience these hormonal disruptions, but it is important to be mindful that they can occur. Overall, while there may be specific circumstances where a ketogenic diet is helpful, it remains a risky approach and cannot yet be recommended as a general approach for treating infertility.

The same is true of intermittent fasting, which involves going without food for periods of time from 16 hours to several days. The theory is that intermittent fasting reduces inflammation and helps boost mitochondrial function, which could therefore improve fertility. We do not yet have good quality research backing up that claim.

To the contrary, the limited studies performed so far suggest that fasting for long periods of time (more than 14 hours per day) is likely to be counterproductive for those trying to conceive, because it disturbs the balance of hormones that control egg development and ovulation.[35] A better approach is to focus on anti-inflammatory strategies that are supported by clear scientific evidence, such as switching to low–glycemic index carbohydrates, avoiding sugar, and adopting a Mediterranean diet.

Do I need to go gluten free?

It has been known for many years that celiac disease can contribute to infertility and recurrent miscarriage. This is likely because the immune reaction to gluten causes nutrient deficiencies and inflammation throughout the body, which can then undermine the ability to get pregnant and carry to term.

More recent research suggests that this link is not limited to women with actual celiac disease—even milder sensitivities to gluten can likely contribute to infertility and miscarriage.[36] From a practical standpoint, this means that it is probably worthwhile eliminating gluten if you have any condition in which inflammation triggered by gluten could be a contributing factor, namely

- unexplained infertility,
- unexplained recurrent miscarriage,
- hypothyroidism, or
- endometriosis.

Celiac disease also has a strong genetic component, so it is worth strictly eliminating gluten if anyone in your family has this condition. You can also order a genetic test to see if you carry a genetic predisposition to celiac disease, known as the HLA-DQ test, which involves sending in a cheek swab for DNA analysis (available from lifextension.com, for example).

Given the number of women who have a reason to avoid gluten while trying to conceive, all recipes in this book are gluten free.

How strictly should I avoid sugar? Are artificial sweeteners better?

In recent years scientists have revealed just how addictive sugar is, activating similar brain pathways as cocaine addiction. This has led many health experts to recommend a "cold-turkey" approach to giving up sugar, eliminating it entirely in order to break the cycle of sugar addiction.

This is a laudable goal, but strictly cutting out sugar can be a major undertaking, given that it is often hidden in unexpected places, such as bacon and salad dressings.[37] For most people, it is likely not necessary to go to the extreme of eliminating all sources of sugar, particularly since fruit contains some sugar yet appears to be associated with improved fertility.

Given that our ultimate goal is balancing blood sugar levels and preventing insulin spikes, what matters most is avoiding major sources of sugar, such as cakes, cookies, candy, sweetened breakfast cereals, ice cream, and flavored yogurts. Limiting these foods to special occasions should be enough to eventually quash sugar cravings, even if you still include some modest sources of sugar, such as whole fruits.

The small amounts of sugar added to foods such as bacon and condiments will not have much impact on blood sugar levels or taste buds, so these hidden sugars are probably not worth worrying about.

Coffee, however, can be a major sugar source. A Starbucks caramel macchiato, for example, can have 32 grams of sugar, equivalent to 8 teaspoons. A better option is to add sweetener yourself, so you can control the amount. A single teaspoon of sugar has 4 grams of sugar, which would not have a major impact on blood glucose levels.

For many people, another major challenge in giving up sugar is finding an alternative to soda. Diet soda is not a good option, because chemical artificial sweeteners appear to wreak havoc with insulin levels in much the same way as sugar.[38] Researchers have also reported a link between diet soda consumption and poor egg and embryo quality.[39] In addition, the artificial sweetener saccharin has been linked to DNA damage in sperm.[40] Rather than switching to diet soda, a better choice is sparkling water flavored with juice such as lemon, lime, pomegranate, or cranberry.

When it comes to baking and desserts, replacing some or all of the sugar in a recipe with natural plant-based sweeteners such as erythritol and monk fruit extract can help reduce the total sugar content. Erythritol is a sugar alcohol that is likely safe from a fertility standpoint but can sometimes cause minor gastrointestinal side effects such as gas and bloating. Monk fruit extract, also known as luo han guo, is another natural sugar alternative that appears to be safer than chemical artificial sweeteners and avoids some of the side effects of erythritol, although some people find the taste unpleasant. Another natural sweetener that can be used occasionally is stevia, but animal studies have raised the possibility that it could interfere with reproductive hormones.[41] For this reason, stevia should not be used on a daily basis.

Is honey or maple syrup better than sugar?

There is a common misconception that using natural sweeteners, such as honey, agave, maple syrup, or dates, is healthier than conventional sugar. In reality, the difference in nutritional content is minimal and all these sweeteners will cause a similar rise in blood sugar and insulin levels.

Ultimately, it is the total amount of sweetener in each portion that matters, not whether it is in the form of honey, maple syrup, or regular sugar. When baking, the best strategy is to reduce the sugar called for by at least one-third and keep portion size small. You can also replace some or all of the sugar in a recipe with erythritol, if tolerated.

An even better alternative is to rely on whole fruit as a sweet snack or dessert. The sugar in fruit will be released more slowly because it is bound together with fiber. In addition, the array of vitamins and antioxidants present in fruit helps compensate for the impact on blood sugar.

Dark chocolate is another good choice, because the total amount of sugar is relatively low, and it is also rich in antioxidants. Research has demonstrated that regular consumption of dark chocolate can help reduce oxidative stress,[42] which we know has a significant impact on egg and sperm quality. To minimize sugar, look for dark chocolate with at least 70 percent cocoa.

How can I put a stop to sugar cravings?

If you are finding it very difficult to cut back on sugar, rest assured that it gets easier with time. As you switch to low–glycemic index carbohydrates, you will have fewer blood sugar crashes that lead to carbohydrate cravings. And taste preferences really do change.[43] When researchers in California asked a group of people to cut out all added sugars and artificial sweeteners for two weeks, 95 percent of participants reported that sugary foods and drinks tasted sweeter or too sweet.[44] The vast majority of participants in the study also reported that sugar cravings stopped within six days.

If you continue to struggle with sugar cravings, consider temporarily avoiding fruit and adding a probiotic supplement, in order to rebalance your gut microbiome. Although this sounds far-fetched, research suggests that the microbes in our gut can help shape our food preferences and cravings, prompting us to eat more of the foods they thrive on.[45]

According to this theory, a healthy gut microbiome leads us to prefer vegetables and other high-fiber foods, whereas an overgrowth of species that metabolize simple sugars, such as yeast, may increase the desire for sugar and refined carbohydrates. By starving yeast and other unwanted species of sugars and building up the population of beneficial microbes, we can put a stop to this vicious cycle, making it much easier to stick to a healthy diet.

If you decide to add a probiotic supplement, one particularly beneficial strain is *Lactobacillus Rhamnosus GG*, found in Culturelle and several other brands. This strain has been demonstrated to suppress the growth of yeast species such as *Candida*,[46] while reducing inflammation and supporting gut health. (See *The Keystone Approach* for more details on how probiotics reduce inflammation.)

How does exercise impact insulin levels and fertility?

Exercise has profound benefits for balancing blood sugar and reducing insulin resistance, in both the short and long term.

After a single bout of moderate-intensity exercise, the ability of muscles to take up glucose from the bloodstream is heightened for at least two days. This is likely because the store of glycogen in muscles gets depleted, so the next time blood sugar rises, the muscles can quickly absorb this excess glucose and store it as glycogen.

Over the long term, regular physical activity also helps the body become more adept at handling glucose and insulin, preventing the high levels of insulin that can disrupt reproductive hormones.[47]

This explains a pattern reported in numerous studies: women who engage in regular, moderate-intensity exercise have improved fertility.[48] This trend is strongest in women who are overweight, have PCOS, or irregular ovulation, but it also applies more generally.[49] In the IVF context, studies have found that physically active women have almost a two-fold higher chance of pregnancy and live birth.[50]

There is a sweet spot, however. Frequent high-intensity exercise appears to cause too much stress for the body, disrupting hormones and thereby compromising fertility.[51] For this reason, athletes have an unusually high rate of ovulation disorders and infertility. It is hard to know what counts as too intense and it may differ between individuals, but you should be able to carry on a conversation while exercising and should not feel completely exhausted afterward.

For women trying to conceive through IVF, it may be necessary to further limit exercise in the weeks before egg retrieval and immediately after embryo transfer. In the lead-up to egg retrieval, ovaries become unusually enlarged and this can make exercise uncomfortable or even painful. There is also a small risk of ovarian torsion, a complication in which the ovary twists around the ligaments that hold it in place, potentially compromising the blood supply.

Although ovarian torsion is very rare, it can be extremely painful and require surgery. One of the main risk factors is sudden movement, particularly turning or twisting motions. Clinics therefore advise women to avoid these types of movements (and yoga inversions) in the weeks before and after egg retrieval, when stimulation medications can result in enlarged ovaries at higher risk of torsion.

Following embryo transfer, most doctors take a conservative approach and recommend rest, but there is very little evidence to go on. In one study, researchers compared the results of 1 hour versus 24 hours of bed rest following embryo transfer. Perhaps somewhat surprisingly, there was a higher rate of embryo implantation in the group that resumed their normal activities after only an hour. Other studies have similarly found no benefit from extended bed rest after embryo transfer.[52]

For men, exercise seems to have very little impact on sperm quality or fertility, either positive or negative. The one exception is cycling, which significantly reduces sperm concentration while increasing the proportion of sperm with abnormal motility and morphology.[53] Cycling appears to pose a particular problem because it involves compression forces and high temperatures, both of which pose a threat to sperm development.[54] Given that it takes at least three months for sperm to mature, regular cycling should be avoided for at least that length of time before IVF or IUI.

Chapter 4

Protein

Goal: Fill one-quarter of your plate with protein

"PROTEIN IS ESSENTIAL for good quality embryos and better egg quality," says Dr. Jeffrey Russell, director of the Delaware Institute for Reproductive Medicine. One of the main benefits of including protein with every meal and snack is keeping blood sugar levels steady. Protein not only slows the release of glucose from carbohydrate-rich foods but also provides greater satiety, so you can reduce the amount of carbohydrates without feeling hungry.

Over time, a moderate- or high-protein diet also improves insulin sensitivity.[55] This means the cells in the body become better at responding to insulin's message to take up glucose from the blood, preventing blood sugar spikes and the resulting hormonal disruptions.

Exactly how much protein do I need?

For fertility purposes, it appears that the optimal amount of protein is at least 25 percent of calories, which amounts to 125 grams for a woman consuming 2000 calories per day. What might this look like in a day?

Breakfast

Omelet with 2 eggs and 1 cup mushrooms = 16 g protein

Lunch

Green salad with 6 ounces chicken breast and ½ cup chickpeas = 60 g protein

Snack

1 cheese stick with 1 apple = 8 g protein

Dinner

6 ounces grilled salmon with 1 cup broccoli and ½ cup brown rice = 46 g protein

Total = 130 grams

A simple way to ensure you get enough protein every day is to choose a protein-rich breakfast (such as eggs, yogurt, chicken sausage, or a protein smoothie) and include a 4- to 6-ounce serving of chicken, fish, or lean meat at lunch and dinner. This serving size is a little larger than the palm of your hand.

It is more difficult to reach the goal of 40 to 50 grams of protein per meal from vegetarian sources, but it can be done by combining some of the following protein-rich foods:

- tofu (40 g per cup)

- edamame (18 g per cup)

- lentils (18 g per cup)

- chickpeas (15 g per cup)

- pinto beans (15 g per cup)

- black-eyed peas (11 g per cup)

- green peas (8 g per cup)

- quinoa (8 g per cup)

- oats (6 g per half cup)

Which proteins are best for fertility?

When it comes to fertility diets, one of the main debates is whether it is better to obtain protein from plant or animal sources. One of the largest studies in this area, the Nurses' Health Study, found that women who obtained more of their protein from vegetarian sources such as soy and beans had a lower risk of ovulatory infertility, which is typically caused by PCOS. Consuming more animal protein, on the other hand, was associated with a higher risk of this specific type of infertility.[56]

One possible explanation for this pattern is that the saturated fat found in meat causes a greater inflammatory response in women with PCOS, as will be discussed later in this chapter. This inflammation further exacerbates the hormonal disruptions involved in PCOS, explaining why animal proteins may pose a problem. We can address this issue by choosing leaner cuts of meat and placing greater emphasis on fish and chicken.

Leaving aside the specific case of ovulatory infertility and looking at fertility more generally, it is clear that the best protein sources for couples trying to conceive are those at the heart of the Mediterranean diet, namely legumes and fish, with some poultry and limited amounts of red meat.

More specifically, numerous studies have found that eating more fish is associated with shorter times to pregnancy for couples trying to conceive naturally and better outcomes in IVF cycles.[57] These better outcomes include a higher number of good-quality embryos and a higher live birth rate.

Fish consumption is also strongly associated with higher sperm quality.[58] In particular, men with higher omega-3 levels typically show improved morphology and a lower percentage of DNA damage.[59]

Studies have also found that legumes are beneficial for fertility, and poultry is either neutral or beneficial. One study reported a higher fertilization rate in IVF when men had a higher intake of poultry.[60] This is likely because chicken is one of the best sources of vitamin B6, which plays a key role in supporting sperm development.

Animal-based proteins have many other fertility benefits too, by virtue of their nutrient density. Fish, poultry, and eggs, for example, are among the best sources of a whole range of vitamins and minerals that are essential to healthy egg and embryo development. This includes vitamin B6, B12, choline, omega-3 fatty acids, selenium, and zinc, which play a vital role in detoxification, reducing inflammation, and preventing oxidative damage to developing eggs and sperm.

TOP SOURCES OF FERTILITY-FRIENDLY VITAMINS AND MINERALS

Vitamin B6	Vitamin B12	Choline	Selenium	Zinc
chickpeas	clams	eggs	brazil nuts	oysters
salmon	sardines	chicken breast	fish	beef
chicken breast	beef	lean beef	pork	lentils
potatoes	tuna	cod	beef	chickpeas
turkey	trout		chicken	pumpkin seeds
banana	salmon		turkey	cashews
ground beef	dairy		eggs	dairy
	eggs			

If you are following a plant-based diet, you will likely need to rely on supplements to get enough choline and omega-3 fatty acids, as discussed further in this chapter. Vegan and vegetarian diets are also typically low in vitamin B6, B12, zinc, and selenium, so it is helpful to choose a prenatal that includes higher amounts of these nutrients. (See www.itstartswiththeegg.com/supplements)

Is it necessary to cut back on red meat?

For women, the research on red meat and fertility is conflicting, with some studies finding a slight benefit and others reporting a negative impact for women undergoing IVF.[61] For men, however, there is more consistent evidence that red meat compromises fertility, resulting in lower sperm count and poorer morphology and motility scores in men who eat more red meat.[62]

This trend is particularly clear in the case of meat that is highly processed or high in saturated fat, such as bacon and fatty cuts of beef. These foods do not need to be completely eliminated, but it is likely best for men to limit red meat to two servings per week and to choose leaner cuts of meat where possible.

Are protein powders fertility friendly?

Protein powders can be a convenient way to reach your daily protein needs, particularly if you are vegetarian or have limited breakfast options because of food sensitivities or allergies. Yet in recent years, protein powders have come under suspicion as a result of tests showing that over half of the best-selling brands contain detectable levels of BPA, and three-quarters have detectable levels of lead, along with other metals such as arsenic and cadmium.

These test results are somewhat concerning but do not necessarily mean that protein powders need to be avoided. Just because these contaminants can be detected in a sample does not mean that the level is high enough to pose a risk to health and fertility.

In the case of lead, for example, the worst-performing protein powder in one of the studies was produced by Vega, who noted that the amount of lead was still far below the stringent California Prop 65 standard and less than the amount commonly found in many plant-based foods, such as cucumbers and spinach.

The fact is that many plants naturally absorb lead from the soil. As a result, plant-based foods and protein sources will contain some lead, but the amount is unlikely to be high enough to pose significant health concerns. Buying products grown and manufactured in countries such as the United States, rather than China, and choosing a brand that regularly tests for lead and other contaminants can minimize any risk. If you are not vegetarian or vegan, it is preferable to choose whey, egg white, or collagen proteins, because these options contain little to no lead or other heavy metals.

Another potential concern with protein powders is the presence of BPA and other similar endocrine disruptors, likely leaching from plastic manufacturing equipment or plastic packaging. This is a problem that is harder to address through careful product selection, because there is no real way to know which brands or types of protein powder are better in this regard.

The possible presence of BPA is simply a price to pay for the convenience of protein powders. If including protein powder helps you stick to a balanced diet, the best solution is to focus on minimizing your overall BPA exposure from other sources, such as canned food and plastic kitchenware. Recent research also suggests that a diet rich in natural sources of folate can help minimize the harmful impact of BPA, so it may be that adding strawberries and leafy greens to a smoothie can to some extent cancel out the potential negative impact of BPA in protein powders.

Why is fish so beneficial for fertility? Can I just take an omega-3 supplement?

Studies have found that couples who consume the most fish typically have the shortest time to pregnancy and higher IVF success rates.[63] One of the likely reasons is that fish is high in vitamin B6, an important nutrient that works together with folate to lower the level of homocysteine.[64] This in turn boosts fertility in a variety of ways, including by reducing inflammation.

Fish is also rich in omega-3 fatty acids, which play a key role in developing eggs and sperm. When researchers measure the levels of omega-3 fatty acids found in the body, there is a clear relationship between higher levels and improved female fertility.[65] In women undergoing fertility treatment at Massachusetts General Hospital, for example, the clinical pregnancy and live birth rate was 8 percent higher for every 1 percent increase in serum omega-3 levels.[66] Other studies have also found a link between levels of omega-3 fatty acids in the bloodstream and IVF success rates.[67]

At least for men, it appears that taking a daily fish oil supplement produces many of the same benefits as consuming seafood, with studies finding a significant reduction in DNA damage in sperm.[68] Yet there has been very little research on fish oil supplements for female fertility. The few studies performed so far have produced conflicting evidence.[69]

Even so, given what is known about the benefits of omega-3 fats, it makes sense for both men and women trying to conceive to ensure they are getting enough. The best source is cold-water fish, such as salmon, sardines, or mackerel, but the next best option is adding a fish oil supplement providing approximately 700 to 1000 milligrams per day of omega 3s.

For vegans, the best omega-3 source is an algae-based EPA and DHA supplement, such as Nordic Naturals Algae Omega. The omega-3 fats found in most plant sources (such as flax seed) have only limited anti-inflammatory effects, and humans cannot effectively convert these fats to EPA or DHA.[70]

Once you are pregnant, an omega-3 supplement becomes even more important, because these fatty acids play a critical role in supporting infant brain development and reducing the risk of preterm birth, as discussed in depth in my pregnancy book, *Brain Health from Birth*.

Is farmed fish safe?

Although farmed fish has a bad reputation, when you choose the right species from reputable suppliers, it can actually be a good choice. From a nutritional standpoint, there is very little difference between farmed and wild salmon, for instance, with farmed possibly having a slight edge due to a higher fat content and therefore a higher concentration of omega-3 fatty acids.[71] In years past, it appeared the high levels of omega-6 fat in farmed salmon was a concern, but this has been dispelled by more recent research showing farmed and wild are closely equivalent. Farmed salmon is also more readily available and affordable than wild salmon, and many people prefer the milder taste.

Farmed fish does pose some concern with respect to antibiotic use and potential environmental harm, but this can be minimized by purchasing from sources such as Costco and WholeFoods, which impose strict standards on suppliers, or buying fish produced in highly regulated countries, such as Iceland, and avoiding that produced in Asia.

As noted by the Monterey Bay Aquarium's Seafood Watch Program, "the environmental impact of fish farming varies widely, depending on the species being farmed, the methods used and where the farm is located. When good practices are used, it's possible to farm seafood in a way that has very little impact to the environment." Seafood Watch, for example, rates farmed branzino from the Mediterranean region as a "Good Alternative."

For more specific advice on seafood available in your area, see https://www.seafoodwatch.org/seafood-recommendations/consumer-guides.

Is the mercury in fish a concern?

Although there are some species of fish that are very high in mercury and should be avoided while trying to conceive, most fresh fish available at the supermarket is safe. The best options are those that are highest in omega-3 fatty acids and lowest in mercury:

- salmon (farmed or wild)
- sardines
- Atlantic mackerel
- herring

See below for a comparison of the mercury levels in other common types of fish.

The main concern with mercury comes from regular consumption of tuna. A small can of albacore tuna has three-quarters of the weekly limit for mercury, and the mercury level in some types of tuna served at sushi restaurants (such as bigeye and bluefin) is higher still. Even the lowest-mercury tuna, canned chunk light, has more than a quarter of the weekly limit of mercury in a small serving. By comparison, the same-size serving of salmon has only 2 percent of the mercury limit. To look up mercury levels for other fish species, consult the Environmental Defense Fund Seafood Selector tool, available online at http://seafood.edf.org/.

VERY LOW MERCURY (3 OR MORE SERVINGS PER WEEK)

Fish	DHA + EPA per 100 g (3.5 oz.)	Mercury (ppm)
Atlantic salmon, farmed	2.1	0.02
Atlantic salmon, wild	1.8	0.05
Herring	1.7	0.06
Sardines	1.5	0.08
Atlantic mackerel	1.2	0.05
Sockeye salmon, wild	1.2	0.04

Farmed trout	1.2	0.03
Coho salmon, wild	1.1	0.04
Atlantic cod	0.12	0.03

MODERATE MERCURY (1 SERVING PER WEEK)

Fish	DHA + EPA per 100 g (3.5 oz.)	Mercury (ppm)
Mackerel, chub	1.8	0.1
Sablefish (black cod)	1.8	0.2
Halibut, from Greenland	1.2	0.2
Sole	0.5	0.09
Flounder	0.5	0.1
Hake	0.5	0.2
Skipjack tuna	0.3	0.2
Tuna, light, canned	0.3	0.1
Tuna, yellowfin, canned	0.3	0.1
Perch	0.3	0.1
Snapper	0.3	0.2
Haddock	0.2	0.2

HIGH MERCURY (1 TO 2 SERVINGS PER MONTH)

Fish	Mercury (ppm)
Halibut, Pacific	0.3
Tuna, albacore, canned	0.3
Grouper	0.4
Bass, Chilean	0.4
Mackerel, Spanish	0.4
Orange roughy	0.5

VERY HIGH MERCURY (AVOID ENTIRELY)

Fish	Mercury (ppm)
Tuna, bluefin	0.8
Swordfish	0.9
Mackerel, king	1.1
Marlin	1.5

Is it safe to eat canned fish?

Although the general advice is to avoid canned food in order to minimize exposure to BPA, many manufacturers have now moved to safer materials for their can linings for seafood. Wild Planet, for example, does not use BPA in their cans. Other brands may still include small amounts of BPA or equivalent chemicals, but the nutritional benefits of eating fish likely outweigh any potential risk, particularly for salmon and sardines. Glass jars and foil pouches are even safer options, and these can be purchased online.

Are eggs helpful for fertility?

Eggs are a fertility superfood because they are among the richest sources of choline, a key nutrient that helps with detoxification, much like folate. A deficiency of choline can in fact produce many of the same effects as a folate deficiency,[72] indicating that it is probably just as important to fertility. Choline is also essential during early pregnancy to support infant brain development, as discussed in detail in my pregnancy book, *Brain Health from Birth*.

Unfortunately, this critical nutrient is rarely found in sufficient amounts in prenatal and multivitamin supplements. Researchers have also found that women are usually deficient in choline unless they eat eggs on a daily basis.[73]

Eggs are uniquely helpful in this context because each egg has one-third of the recommended daily intake of choline. Specifically, the recommended daily intake is 450 mg per day; an egg has approximately 150 mg of choline. A six-ounce serving of chicken breast, lean beef, or cod also has approximately 140 mg, allowing you to reach the daily goal of 450 mg with two eggs for breakfast and a serving of animal protein for lunch or dinner, for example.

Liver is another good source of choline, but it is too high in vitamin A to consume regularly in the lead-up to pregnancy. High levels of vitamin A during pregnancy can potentially increase the risk of birth defects, so the recommended upper limit is 10,000 IU per day. A single three-ounce serving of liver contains 26,000 IU of vitamin A. This amount can be eaten occasionally but not on a daily basis. Regular consumption of cod liver oil is not recommended for the same reason.

For vegetarians and vegans, it is much more difficult to get sufficient choline. The highest plant-based sources of choline include soybeans, quinoa, kidney beans, broccoli, and Brussels sprouts. Each of these sources only provides 30 to 50 mg per serving, however, so a supplement is typically necessary to avoid a deficiency. (Look for 350 to 500 mg of choline bitartrate.)

Is soy good or bad for fertility?

For many years, women trying to conceive have been advised to avoid soy, on the theory that it may disrupt the delicate balance of reproductive hormones. Yet there is little evidence backing up this contention.[74] To the contrary, the most recent studies suggest that soy may actually be beneficial for fertility.

As one example, researchers at the Harvard School of Public Health reported a significantly higher chance of live birth in women who consumed more soy during fertility treatment.[75] Other researchers have reported positive results from giving women soy phytoestrogen supplements during IVF, with a higher chance of implantation, pregnancy, and live birth.[76]

Soy also seems to be helpful for women trying to conceive naturally, since it is associated with a lower risk of ovulatory infertility.[77] This could be because soy contains compounds that may improve insulin resistance in women with PCOS.[78]

The possibility has been raised that the phytoestrogens present in soy could be problematic for men, but this does not seem to be supported by the evidence. One early study suggested that very high soy consumption by men could reduce sperm concentration slightly, without influencing other measures of sperm quality such as motility and morphology.[79] More recent studies have found no impact on any measure of sperm quality and no impact on IVF success rates in men who consume the most soy.[80]

Even though soy appears to be beneficial for most people trying to conceive, the question remains whether some people may benefit from excluding soy, because of thyroid or other autoimmune conditions.

One of the long-standing concerns over soy in the fertility context is the potential to interfere with thyroid function. This problem was first flagged by animal studies and reports of thyroid problems occurring in babies exclusively fed with soy formula. Yet soy seems to have much less impact on thyroid function in the real world. In adults consuming soy as part of a normal diet, there is little to no impact on the levels of T3 or T4 thyroid hormones.[81] Soy intake may be associated with a slightly higher TSH level, but it is not clear that this has any practical significance.[82]

If soy does impact thyroid function, this could possibly be the result of activating the immune response in those who already have thyroid autoimmunity and who have a specific immune sensitivity to soybeans.[83] More research is needed in this area, but it may be worth avoiding soy out of an abundance of caution if you have high levels of thyroid antibodies (or any other autoimmune disease). That said, there are other foods that are probably more important to strictly eliminate in order to address thyroid autoimmunity—namely wheat, corn, and dairy. Those specific foods appear to trigger a significantly greater immune response against the thyroid.[84]

Is dairy good or bad for fertility?

So far, the research indicates that dairy is either neutral or slightly beneficial for fertility. Among women trying to conceive naturally, studies have found that greater consumption of dairy is associated with a shorter time to pregnancy.[85] A recent study of women undergoing IVF also found a higher live birth rate among those who consume the most dairy.[86]

Yet there are nuances to this, with some research drawing a distinction between different types of dairy. The Nurses' Health Study, for example, found that full-fat dairy was beneficial for women trying to conceive, whereas low-fat dairy was associated with higher odds of ovulatory infertility. This difference was not seen in a more recent, larger study,[87] but if low-fat dairy really is problematic for women, it is likely because it has more impact on insulin levels.

On the other hand, it appears that low-fat dairy is better for men than higher-fat dairy.[88] One study found that low-fat milk intake was associated with higher sperm concentration and progressive motility, whereas cheese intake was associated with lower sperm concentration, count, and progressive motility.[89] This could be because saturated fat has a particularly negative impact on sperm quality, as discussed further below.

Although dairy as a general rule is not harmful for fertility, it is a very common allergen, and for some individuals, an immune reaction to dairy could be inflammatory. For this reason, if you suspect that inflammation could be involved in your fertility issues, it may be worth excluding all dairy for two weeks and then seeing how you feel when you reintroduce it. If dairy causes gastrointestinal symptoms, sinus congestion, cough, or skin irritation, that suggests you could be better off eliminating dairy long term.

Avoiding dairy may also be particularly helpful for those with autoimmune conditions, such as hypothyroidism. Dr. Izabella Wentz, author of *Hashimoto's Protocol*, notes that "second only to gluten, dairy is one of the most problematic foods for people with Hashimoto's, and I have found that eliminating these two foods from the diet can have the most profound effect on bringing a thyroid disorder into remission."

How can diet impact inflammation?

The term "inflammation" refers to the body's natural response to injury or infection. In the right time and place, this immune activity serves an important function. But all too often, chronic low-grade inflammation occurs throughout the body, with the immune system responding inappropriately and inflicting collateral damage. New research is showing just how much negative impact this can have on fertility.

For example, in women with higher levels of inflammation level before IVF, fewer eggs make it to the 3-day embryo stage.[90] Studies have also linked excessive inflammation to unexplained infertility and recurrent miscarriage.[91]

Fortunately, inflammation is something we have the power to change. As discussed in detail in *It Starts with the Egg*, reducing exposure to toxins such as phthalates can make a big difference, as can adding supplements such as N-acetylcysteine. Diet can also have a profound impact.

Food allergies are likely a major contributor to inflammation, with gluten and dairy as the most common culprits. Another way in which diet impacts inflammation is by altering gut health. The microbiome is the community of microbes that lives in our gastrointestinal system and can have a major influence on the immune system. More than 70 percent of our immune system resides in our gut, where it receives constant signals from the microbes that reside there. Beneficial microbes, which typically thrive when we follow a diet emphasizing fiber-rich plants, send signals to the immune system that calm inflammation and prevent autoimmunity.

In contrast, sugar, saturated fat, and antibiotics can disrupt the balance of species in the microbiome, compromising gut health and setting the stage for the modern epidemic of autoimmune and inflammatory conditions, including asthma, eczema, allergies, and thyroid conditions. (For more detail on this topic, see my autoimmune diet book, *The Keystone Approach*.)

In short, the first steps to reducing inflammation through diet have already been covered: reducing sugar and increasing fiber. Choosing vegetables and legumes over sugar and refined starches not only helps balance blood sugar levels and therefore balance hormones but can also make a big difference to inflammation levels by altering the gut microbiome.

Yet these are not the only dietary strategies we have to regulate unwanted immune activity. There is now a vast body of research showing that the specific types of fat and oil emphasized in the Mediterranean diet can also help quash inflammation, as the next chapter explains.[92]

Chapter 5

Fats and Oils

Goal: Add 1 to 2 servings of healthy fats

THE MEDITERRANEAN DIET heavily emphasizes olive oil, nuts, and fish, all of which provide beneficial fatty acids. Olive oil, in particular, is likely a major reason why the Mediterranean diet is so helpful for fertility, because it is highly anti-inflammatory.[93] After just a single meal including extra-virgin olive oil, a reduction in inflammatory markers and oxidative stress can be detected in the bloodstream.[94] When consumed regularly, this translates into improved symptoms of inflammatory diseases.[95]

The main type of fat found in olive oil is a monounsaturated fat called oleic acid. Other foods rich in monounsaturated fats include nuts, avocados, and high-oleic safflower oil. All these fat sources are likely very helpful for fertility, with studies finding a link between higher levels of monounsaturated fats and shorter time to pregnancy.[96]

In women undergoing IVF, higher levels of oleic acid also seem to be associated with a higher number of mature eggs and improved embryo quality.[97] One IVF study found that women who had a greater intake of monounsaturated fat had three times higher odds of live birth after embryo transfer.[98]

Likely due in part to their high concentration of monounsaturated fats, nuts are another fertility superfood. This benefit is particularly clear for men, with studies linking greater nut consumption to significantly higher sperm quality.[99] In a controlled study published in 2018, one group of men were told to consume at least 60 grams of a mixture of nuts every day for 14 weeks, while the control group consumed no nuts. At the end of the trial, the men who had eaten nuts on a daily basis showed significantly higher scores for sperm count, motility, and morphology.[100] There was also a clear reduction in sperm DNA fragmentation.

In that study, the men consumed about two small handfuls per day of a combination of almonds, walnuts, and hazelnuts. These nuts are particularly beneficial because they are high in monounsaturated fats and low in saturated fat. Other nuts with a high proportion of healthy fats include pecans, peanuts, and pistachios. Cashews and macadamias are less beneficial because they have a lower percentage of monounsaturated fat and more saturated fat.

Omega-3 fats, found in fish, are also particularly good at quashing inflammation and therefore supporting egg and sperm quality. In fact, the combination of omega-3 fatty acids and a diet emphasizing olive oil is especially powerful. Studies have found that when a combination of fish oil and olive oil is compared to a fish oil supplement alone, the combination lowers inflammation much more effectively.[101]

This combination has now been tested in the fertility context, with promising results. In a double-blind, controlled study published in 2020, couples were given olive oil, omega-3 fatty acids, and vitamin D for six weeks before IVF, in an attempt to replicate some of the benefits of a Mediterranean diet. This combination appeared to significantly improve embryo quality.[102]

Is coconut oil good for fertility?

With the rise of the paleo diet in recent years, there has been a growing trend of regarding coconut oil, ghee, and other animal fats as healthy, because they are less processed than refined vegetable oils. The latest scientific research suggests that this is a mistake and that coconut oil, ghee, palm oil, lard, and other saturated fats are actually highly inflammatory.[103]

Minimizing these fats may be just as important to fertility as including more of the healthy monounsaturated fats. In fact, the low level of saturated fat in the Mediterranean diet may be part of the explanation for its fertility benefits.

Scientists have discovered that one of the ways saturated fat triggers inflammation is by forming "lipid rafts" that transport bacterial toxins across the gut barrier. These toxins then provoke the immune system, causing a wave of inflammation throughout the body.[104] Research has found that coconut oil is one of the worst culprits from this perspective, sparking high levels of inflammation.[105]

Studies on the impact of saturated fat on female fertility are just beginning, but so far we know that women with higher levels of saturated fat in their bloodstream appear to produce fewer mature eggs in IVF cycles and end up with a lower percentage of good-quality embryos.[106]

Interestingly, it seems that having higher levels of oleic acid (from olive oil) and omega-3 fats (from fish) can to some extent cancel out the harmful impact of saturated fat on egg and embryo quality.[107]

What is the impact of saturated fat on sperm quality?

It is beyond question that saturated fat is harmful for male fertility. Numerous studies have linked high intake of saturated fat with lower sperm count and sperm concentration.[108] In one of these studies, the men with the highest intake of saturated fat had a 40 percent lower sperm count.[109] This likely explains the trends discussed earlier of reduced fertility among men with high intakes of red meat, processed meat, and full-fat dairy.[110]

That does not mean these foods need to be eliminated completely, but it is worth relying more heavily on chicken, fish, or vegetarian proteins, while minimizing cheese, fatty meats, and other foods high in saturated fat. It also means not cooking with saturated fats, such as coconut oil, ghee, butter, lard, and palm oil, and instead using olive oil, avocado oil, or high-oleic safflower oil.

The combination of lowering saturated fat while increasing monounsaturated fats can significantly improve overall sperm quality.[111] This is likely a major reason why the Mediterranean diet is associated with significantly improved male fertility and improved scores of sperm motility and morphology.[112]

How does fat intake affect PCOS?

Many women with PCOS are encouraged to follow ketogenic or very low-carbohydrate diets that are rich in saturated fat. The latest research suggests this is counterproductive, because the spike in inflammation caused by saturated fat appears to be more extreme in women with PCOS and has more extreme consequences.[113]

In 2020, researchers demonstrated that when women with PCOS consume a meal with saturated fat, they have a rapid increase in inflammatory markers, much greater than seen in healthy women.[114] This is a big problem because higher levels of inflammation can worsen insulin resistance and increase testosterone in women with PCOS.[115] In short, saturated fat may exacerbate the hormonal disruptions that cause infertility in women with PCOS. Reducing fats such as coconut oil, palm oil, and animal fats is likely to be particularly helpful for this condition.

Women with PCOS are also likely to derive even greater benefit from emphasizing the fats at the core of the Mediterranean diet, such as olive oil and omega-3 fatty acids. Researchers have demonstrated that omega-3 fats can improve insulin resistance and inflammation in women with PCOS.[116] This would be expected to improve reproductive hormones and therefore fertility.

Chapter 6

The Non-Toxic Kitchen

ONE OF THE most surprising patterns to emerge in fertility research over the past several decades is the impact of common chemicals on egg and sperm quality. As explained in more detail in *It Starts with the Egg*, this research provides a clear impetus to reduce plastic in the kitchen and switch to safer materials, such as stainless steel and glass. Yet it is not necessary to completely eliminate plastic—rather, the focus should be on replacing those items that are more likely to transfer chemicals to food and drinks. This includes:

- Reusable food storage containers
- Bowls used in the microwave
- Reusable water bottles and cups
- Plastic tea kettles
- Colanders
- Blender containers that have been used with hot soups

Beyond these high-priority items, there are many grey areas and circumstances where continuing to use plastic is the most practical choice, such as water filters and cutting boards. This chapter answers some of the common questions you may have about these grey areas, to help you strike the right balance between chemical safety and practicality in the kitchen.

Can I use nonstick pans?

The concern with nonstick pans comes from the fluorinated chemicals that are used to create a smooth and durable surface. We do not yet know what impact these chemicals have on fertility, but we do know they disrupt hormone activity and accumulate in the body over time, raising serious concerns. One of the worst of the nonstick chemicals, known as PFOA, has now been phased out, but many brands of cookware have replaced it with similar chemicals that may not be any better.

The safest cookware materials are cast iron and stainless steel. It is best to rely on these types of pots and pans as much as possible, but when you do need a nonstick surface, it is reasonable to use a ceramic nonstick pan, such as those made by GreenPan. This safer type of nonstick surface is not as long lasting as Teflon, but you can prolong the life by avoiding high heat and sudden temperature changes and washing by hand. It is also best to use ventilation when cooking with any nonstick pans and to replace pans when the surface becomes scratched or damaged.

For recommendations on specific cookware brands, see www.itstartswiththeegg.com/non-toxic-cookware

What can I use instead of nonstick muffin pans and baking trays?

The best option is to use stainless steel baking sheets or muffin pans. These are difficult to find in stores but can be ordered online (see itstartswiththeegg.com/non-toxic-cookware). The next best option is aluminum. Although there is some controversy over the health risks of aluminum, we absorb only a very small percentage of any aluminum ingested. Although minimizing the use of aluminum may be preferred, it is not our top priority, and this material is likely safer than most brands of nonstick cookware.

Ovenproof glass bakeware, such as Pyrex, is another good option. Silicone muffin pans and baking sheet liners should be avoided, because silicone can release chemicals called siloxanes when heated for prolonged periods of time. We do not yet know what risks, if any, these chemicals pose, but the most cautious approach is to avoid them.

Can I store dry goods, such as rice and flour, in plastic containers?

Yes. There is little risk of chemicals leaching into dry goods, particularly with a safer plastic such as polypropylene.

What is the best material for cutting boards?

The different materials used for cutting boards have their own advantages and disadvantages, but plastic cutting boards are a good option. From a chemical standpoint, the safest material is glass, but glass cutting boards can be unpleasant to use and over time will reduce the sharpness of knives. Wooden cutting boards are nontoxic but can be difficult to sanitize and have a limited lifespan. Bamboo cutting boards are not recommended because the adhesives used to hold the fibers together can contain a cocktail of chemicals.

Polypropylene plastic cutting boards are likely the best compromise between safety and practicality. Polypropylene is one of the safest types of plastic and when used for cutting boards, it will be unlikely to transfer any chemicals to food given the limited contact time.

What about canned drinks and bottled water?

Canned drinks are likely to contain BPA and other similar chemicals and should be avoided when possible. Although brands such as La Croix have switched to BPA-free cans, there is little information available about the new materials being used. Buying drinks in glass bottles is a better alternative.

When glass isn't an option, it is likely safer to buy drinks in plastic bottles rather than cans, because the type of plastic used in single-use water bottles is not normally high in BPA or phthalates. Nevertheless, some degree of chemical leaching may still occur, and it is not recommended to rely on plastic bottled water on a daily basis. The best option for daily drinking water is filtered tap water. Even if a water filter contains some plastic parts, the water is typically not in contact with the plastic for a long period of time. (For recommended brands, see itstartswiththeegg.com/purging-plastics/water-filters.)

My blender container is plastic. Is this a concern?

Currently, most high-end blender makers use a type of plastic called Tritan copolyester for their containers. Although it does not contain BPA and is relatively safe for cool or room-temperature ingredients, Tritan has been found to leach another harmful chemical, Fluorene-9-bisphenol, when in contact with hot liquids. For blending hot soups, a better option is to use a stainless-steel immersion blender or a blender with a glass or stainless-steel container. At the time of writing, Vitamix and Nutri Ninja are available with stainless steel containers.

If you have previously used your plastic blender with hot ingredients or washed it in the dishwasher, it is best to contact the manufacturer for a replacement container.

Can I use Ziploc bags for freezing food?

If budget and freezer space permits, the safest option is to freeze food in glass storage containers. Many brands are freezer safe, including Pyrex, Ikea, and Anchor-Hocking. Glass containers can be bulky, however, so there may be times when it is more practical to use Ziploc bags. Doing so is not a major concern, but it is important to allow food to fully cool before transferring to plastic. Reusable silicone freezer bags are also available and this material is likely preferable to single-use Ziploc bags.

Can I use cling film to prevent splattering in the microwave?

Using cling film in the microwave is not recommended, particularly if it comes into direct contact with hot food. A better alternative is a glass microwave plate cover.

For more recommendations on non-toxic kitchenware, see www.itstartswiththeegg.com/purging-plastics

Part II
Fertility-Friendly Recipes

Recipes

Main Dishes

Breakfasts

BANANA PANCAKES

Serves 2

INGREDIENTS

2 ripe bananas

¼ cup rolled oats

2 large eggs

1 tablespoon oil

½ teaspoon pure vanilla extract

½ teaspoon baking powder

¼ teaspoon ground cinnamon

Combine all the ingredients in a blender or food processor and blend until smooth. Heat a nonstick pan over medium-low heat. Pour the batter into the pan to form 3- to 4-inch pancakes. Cook for 3 to 4 minutes per side.

ALMOND FLOUR PANCAKES

Serves 2

2 large eggs plus 1 egg white

2 tablespoons water or milk of choice

1 tablespoon avocado oil

¾ cup almond flour (not almond meal)

1 tablespoon coconut flour

1 teaspoon sugar or erythritol

½ teaspoon baking powder

½ teaspoon pure vanilla extract

Pinch salt

In a bowl or measuring jug, beat the eggs and water. Add the remaining ingredients and whisk to form a smooth batter. The mixture should be the consistency of regular pancake batter. Add 1 to 2 tablespoons of additional water or almond flour if needed. Heat a nonstick pan over medium-low heat. Pour the batter into the pan to form 3- to 4-inch pancakes. Cover and cook for 2 minutes per side.

BUTTERNUT SQUASH PANCAKES

Serves 2

INGREDIENTS

- **2** large eggs
- **1** cup cooked butternut squash
- **1** tablespoon maple syrup or erythritol
- **½** cup gluten-free flour
- **3** tablespoons coconut flour
- **1** teaspoon pure vanilla extract
- **1** teaspoon baking powder
- **¼** teaspoon ground cinnamon

Combine all the ingredients in a blender and blend until smooth. Heat a nonstick pan over medium-low heat. Pour the batter into the pan to form 3- to 4-inch pancakes and cook for 2 minutes or until small bubbles appear. Flip and cook for an additional 1 to 2 minutes.

SMOKED SALMON AND LEEK FRITTATA

Serves 2 to 4

INGREDIENTS

1 tablespoon olive oil

1 medium to large leek, sliced and thoroughly washed

8 large eggs

½ teaspoon salt

1 tablespoon chopped fresh dill or parsley

4 ounces smoked salmon, cut into large flakes

Combine the olive oil and leek in an oven-safe skillet over medium heat. Cover and cook for 8 minutes or until the leek softens. In a large bowl, whisk the eggs, salt, and dill. Distribute the salmon flakes over the leeks in the pan and then pour the egg mixture on top. Cook over medium heat for 5 minutes, until only the center is liquid. In the meantime, preheat the broiler. Place the pan under the broiler until the frittata is cooked through, 3 to 5 minutes. Allow to cool slightly before slicing.

HAM AND MUSHROOM EGG MUFFINS

Serves 2

INGREDIENTS

5 large eggs

½ teaspoon salt

¼ teaspoon black pepper

⅓ cup chopped ham

⅓ cup chopped mushrooms

⅓ cup grated cheese (optional)

Preheat the oven to 400°F (200°C). In a large measuring jug, whisk the eggs, salt, and pepper. Grease 6 cups of a muffin pan and distribute the ham, mushrooms, and cheese (if using) between the muffin cups. Pour the egg mixture on top and stir to combine with the ham and mushrooms. Bake for 12 to 15 minutes or until set.

LOW-CARB SOFT WHITE BREAD

Makes 1 loaf *Recipe inspired by Maya Krampf*

INGREDIENTS

12 large egg whites, at room temperature

¼ teaspoon cream of tartar

¼ cup coconut flour

1 cup blanched almond flour

2 teaspoons baking powder

¼ teaspoon salt

5 tablespoons avocado or safflower oil

1 tablespoon sugar, erythritol, or monk fruit extract

2 teaspoons psyllium husk

Preheat the oven to 325°F (165°C). Grease a (8- by 4-inch) loaf pan.

Use a hand mixer to beat the egg whites and cream of tartar until stiff peaks form. In a separate bowl, combine the coconut flour, almond flour, baking powder, salt, oil, sweetener, and psyllium husk. Add one-quarter of the egg whites. Use the hand mixer to combine. Gently fold in the remaining egg whites.

Pour the mixture into the loaf pan. Bake for 1 hour 15 minutes, until the top is firm. Cover with foil halfway through baking to prevent the top from becoming too brown while the middle cooks through. Allow the bread to cool before removing from the pan and slicing.

COCONUT FLOUR APPLE MUFFINS

Serves 10

INGREDIENTS

4 large eggs

¼ cup avocado or safflower oil

2 to **3** tablespoons honey

2 teaspoons pure vanilla extract

½ cup coconut flour

2 tablespoons cornstarch

1 teaspoon baking powder

2 teaspoons ground cinnamon

1 apple, peeled and diced

Preheat the oven to 400°F (200°C). Grease 10 cups of a muffin tin.

With an electric hand mixer, beat the eggs with the oil, honey, and vanilla until frothy. In a separate bowl or measuring jug, combine the coconut flour, cornstarch, baking powder, and cinnamon. Add the diced apple to the dry ingredients, and then combine with the wet ingredients, stirring until just combined. Scoop the batter into the muffin cups. Transfer to the oven and immediately lower the temperature to 375°F (190°C). Bake for 12 minutes or until just firm in the center.

BLUEBERRY PROTEIN SMOOTHIE

Serves 1

INGREDIENTS

2 to **3** scoops collagen peptide powder

½ cup water or milk of choice

½ cup frozen blueberries

½ banana

½ cup crushed ice

1 tablespoon olive or avocado oil

Mix the collagen powder and water in a glass. Transfer to a blender and combine with the remaining ingredients. Blend until smooth.

GREEN PROTEIN SMOOTHIE

Serves 1

INGREDIENTS

2 to **3** scoops collagen peptide powder

¾ cup water

3 to **5** kale leaves or handful of spinach

½ avocado

½ cup crushed ice

Juice of ½ lime

Handful fresh parsley, basil, mint, or a combination

½ cup diced honeydew melon

Mix the collagen powder and water in a glass. Transfer to a blender and combine with the remaining ingredients. Blend until smooth.

APPLE AND SAGE CHICKEN SAUSAGE

Serves 6

INGREDIENTS

2 pounds ground chicken

1 peeled apple, finely diced

2 fresh sage leaves, finely chopped, or 1 teaspoon dried

1 teaspoon sea salt

2 tablespoons olive oil

1 to **2** teaspoons honey or maple syrup (optional)

Preheat the oven to 425°F (220°C). Line a rimmed baking sheet with foil.

In a large bowl, mix together all the ingredients and then shape into patties about 2 inches wide. Bake on the baking sheet for 12 to 15 minutes. Alternatively, pan-fry in olive oil for 3 minutes per side.

AMERICAN BREAKFAST SAUSAGE

Serves 6

INGREDIENTS

2 pounds lean ground beef

1 tablespoon olive oil

1 teaspoon sea salt

1 teaspoon dried sage

¼ teaspoon dried marjoram

1 tablespoon maple syrup (optional)

Preheat the oven to 425°F (220°C). In a large bowl, mix together all the ingredients and then shape into patties about 2 inches wide. Bake on a baking sheet for 12 to 15 minutes. Alternatively, pan-fry in olive oil for 3 minutes per side.

CHIA PROTEIN PUDDING

Serves 1

INGREDIENTS

½ cup water or milk of choice

2 scoops collagen peptide powder

2 tablespoons chia seeds

1 tablespoon nut butter or sunflower seed butter (optional)

Fresh, frozen, or dried berries (optional)

2 tablespoons unsweetened shredded coconut (optional)

In a small bowl or cup, combine the water and collagen powder, stirring to dissolve. Add the chia seeds, stir, and then refrigerate overnight. When ready to serve, top with your choice of nut butter, berries, and dried coconut.

FLAX PORRIDGE

Serves 1

INGREDIENTS

2 tablespoons freshly ground flax seeds

½ cup boiling water

2 tablespoons hemp hearts

2 tablespoons unsweetened shredded coconut

2 tablespoons collagen peptide powder

¼ teaspoon ground cinnamon

½ tablespoon avocado oil (optional)

Fresh, frozen, or dried berries (optional)

Chopped nuts (optional)

Combine the ground flax seeds and boiling water in a bowl. Add the hemp hearts, coconut, collagen peptide powder, cinnamon, and oil (if using) and stir until well combined. Add additional water or a milk of your choice if needed and top with berries or chopped nuts (if using).

CHICKEN, KALE, AND BUTTERNUT SQUASH HASH

Serves 1

INGREDIENTS

3 large kale leaves

4 to **6** ounces cooked chicken breast, cubed

2 tablespoons avocado oil

¼ teaspoon salt

Pinch poultry seasoning

¼ cup water

1 cup roasted butternut squash

¼ cup chopped fresh parsley

Remove the center ribs from the kale and chop the leaves. Fry the chicken in the avocado oil until lightly browned and then transfer to a plate. To the same pan, add the kale, salt, poultry seasoning, and water. Add the butternut squash (and any other leftover cooked vegetables you have on hand). Cover and cook for 3 minutes. Return the chicken to the pan, along with the parsley, and toss to combine.

Soups and Salads

COLORADO SOUP

Serves 4

INGREDIENTS

⅓ red cabbage

1 large carrot, peeled and sliced

½ onion, finely chopped

1 garlic clove, minced

1 cup cooked black-eyed peas or white beans

2 cups low-sodium chicken broth or water

12 ounces chicken sausage

1 teaspoon salt

1 teaspoon sugar or erythritol (optional)

2 tablespoons tomato pasta sauce (optional)

Remove any damaged outer leaves and core from the cabbage. Chop into 1-inch pieces. Transfer the cabbage to a large pot, along with the carrot, onion, garlic, beans, and chicken broth. Add extra water if needed to cover the vegetables. Simmer over medium heat for 10 minutes or until the cabbage is tender. Cut the chicken sausage in half lengthways and then into half circles, approximately ½ inch thick. Add the sausage to the soup and simmer for 5 minutes. Taste and adjust the seasoning, adding the salt and sweetener or tomato sauce, if desired.

QUICK CHICKEN AND LEEK SOUP

Serves 2 to 4

INGREDIENTS

2 large leeks

1 medium onion, chopped

1 large carrot, chopped

1 celery stalk, chopped

2 tablespoons olive oil

½ teaspoon dried sage

2 cups low-sodium chicken broth

1 rotisserie chicken, meat removed from bones and diced

Salt

Cut the white and light-green parts of the leeks into half-inch rings. Rinse thoroughly and drain. In a large pot over medium-high heat, cook the leeks, onion, carrot, and celery in the olive oil for 5 minutes. Add the dried sage and broth and bring to the boil. After 5 to 10 minutes, when the vegetables are tender, add the chicken and salt to taste. Lower the heat and simmer for 5 minutes.

CLASSIC GREEK SALAD

Serves 4

INGREDIENTS

1 small container cherry tomatoes, halved

1 English cucumber, sliced into half circles

1½ cups cooked chickpeas

½ cup pitted Kalamata olives, diced

½ small red onion, diced

⅓ cup olive oil

2 tablespoons red wine vinegar

1 teaspoon dried oregano

½ teaspoon salt

In a large bowl, combine the tomatoes, cucumber, chickpeas, olives, and onion. In a separate bowl, whisk together the olive oil, vinegar, oregano, and salt. Pour the dressing over the salad and toss to combine. Allow to stand for 30 minutes before serving.

PERFECT BRINED ROAST CHICKEN BREASTS FOR SALADS

Serves 6

INGREDIENTS

2 tablespoons salt

1 tablespoon fresh rosemary

1 teaspoon dried thyme

½ cup boiling water

2 cups ice water

3 large chicken breasts

Olive oil

Brining chicken allows it to retain its flavor and moisture when stored in the refrigerator or freezer. To prepare the brine, combine the salt, rosemary, and thyme in the boiling water. In a large glass bowl, mix the salt solution with the ice water. Add the chicken breasts then cover and refrigerate for 2 to 12 hours. (If brining for more than 3 hours, only use 1½ tablespoons of salt.)

When ready to cook the chicken, preheat the oven to 425°F (220°C). Rinse then dry the chicken with paper towels. Coat lightly with olive oil and roast for 17 to 20 minutes or until cooked through. Alternatively, grill or broil until cooked through.

CALIFORNIAN CHICKEN SALAD

Serves 2

INGREDIENTS

2 to **3** tablespoons mayonnaise

1 tablespoon olive oil

1 tablespoon freshly squeezed lemon juice

2 roast chicken breasts, cubed

½ cup black or red grapes, halved

2 celery stalks, sliced

5 basil leaves, sliced into ribbons

½ avocado, diced

In a large bowl, whisk together the mayonnaise, oil, and lemon juice. Add the chicken, grapes, and celery, and stir to combine. Gently stir in the basil and avocado.

ARUGULA, AVOCADO, AND CHICKEN SALAD

Serves 2

INGREDIENTS

Juice of **½** lemon

1 teaspoon maple syrup

2 tablespoons extra-virgin olive oil

½ teaspoon salt

1 package arugula/rocket, or baby kale or spinach

1 avocado, cubed

1 roast chicken breast, shredded or cubed

In a small bowl, whisk together the lemon juice, maple syrup, olive oil, and salt. Divide the arugula, avocado, and chicken between two large bowls. Pour the dressing over the salad and toss to combine.

SALMON SALAD WRAP

Serves 1

INGREDIENTS

½ avocado, mashed

1 tablespoon mayonnaise

½ scallion, finely chopped

Squeeze lemon juice

1 teaspoon olive oil

1 (6-ounce) can salmon, drained

½ celery stalk, chopped

In a small bowl, combine the avocado, mayonnaise, scallion, lemon juice, and olive oil. Lightly mash the salmon and add to the dressing along with the chopped celery. Mix to combine.

Enjoy as is; wrap in a collard, kale, or lettuce leaf; or use as a dip for crackers or celery sticks (omitting the celery from the salmon mixture).

KALE SALAD WITH APPLES AND PECANS

Serves 2 to 4

INGREDIENTS

2 tablespoons olive oil

Juice of **½** lemon

2 teaspoons maple syrup

½ teaspoon salt

6 large kale leaves

½ apple

½ cup pecans

Whisk together the olive oil, lemon juice, maple syrup, and salt. Cut each kale leaf lengthwise to remove the tough rib, then stack the leaves and slice into thin ribbons. Transfer the kale to a salad bowl and toss to combine with the dressing. Allow to sit for at least 15 minutes. When ready to serve, slice the apples and toast the pecans in a dry pan over medium heat until fragrant. Add the apples and pecans to the kale and toss to combine.

CAJUN AVOCADO SHRIMP SALAD

Serves 2

INGREDIENTS

1 pound large shrimp, peeled and deveined

4 tablespoons olive oil

Juice of **2** limes

1 teaspoon salt

½ teaspoon Cajun seasoning

½ head romaine lettuce

1 avocado

½ cup cherry tomatoes, halved

¼ cup chopped fresh cilantro

If the shrimp are frozen, thaw in a bowl of cold water for approximately 30 minutes. Preheat the oven to 400°F (200°C). In a small bowl, combine the olive oil, lime juice, salt, and Cajun seasoning (this seasoning blend can be substituted with a combination of onion powder, garlic powder, paprika, and cayenne pepper).

Transfer the shrimp to a rimmed baking sheet and pour half the dressing on top, reserving the remainder for the salad. Toss the shrimp to coat evenly with dressing and then roast for 6 to 8 minutes, until just pink and firm.

Rinse and chop the lettuce. In a large salad bowl, combine the lettuce, avocado, tomatoes, cilantro, and remaining dressing. Toss to combine. Top with the roasted shrimp.

BLACK-EYED PEA SALAD

Serves 2 to 4

½ pound dry black-eyed peas, or 3 cups cooked

1 large tomato, diced

½ medium red onion, finely chopped

1 red bell pepper, finely chopped

1 scallion, finely chopped

¼ cup chopped fresh cilantro or parsley

¼ cup avocado, safflower, or light olive oil

3 tablespoons white wine vinegar

½ teaspoon sugar or erythritol (optional)

1 teaspoon salt

½ teaspoon ground coriander

Soak the black-eyed peas for at least 8 hours in a glass bowl filled with water. To cook the beans, simmer them in a pot of boiling water for 45 minutes to an hour or until tender. Alternatively, pressure cook them for 30 minutes and allow 10 minutes for natural release. Allow the beans to cool for an additional 30 minutes before assembling the salad.

In a large glass bowl, combine the black-eyed peas, tomato, onion, bell pepper, scallion, and cilantro. To prepare the dressing, whisk together the oil, vinegar, sweetener (if using), salt, and ground coriander. Pour the dressing over the salad and toss to combine.

TACO SALAD

Serves 2

INGREDIENTS

1 tablespoon avocado oil

½ pound lean ground beef

1 teaspoon granulated garlic

1 teaspoon onion powder

1 teaspoon salt

½ teaspoon ground cumin

½ teaspoon black pepper

1 cup cooked black beans

2 small heads romaine lettuce, chopped

1 cup cherry tomatoes, halved

⅓ cup salsa

For the guacamole

Juice of **1** lime, plus more if needed

1 tablespoon avocado oil

½ teaspoon salt

1 scallion, finely chopped

1 tablespoon chopped fresh cilantro, plus more if needed

1 avocado, diced

Heat the oil in a large pan over medium heat. Add the beef, breaking it up with a spatula or wooden spoon. Sprinkle with the granulated garlic, onion powder, salt, cumin, and pepper (or use taco seasoning mix). Add the black beans. Continue breaking up the meat and stirring occasionally until the meat is lightly browned and any liquid has evaporated, 5 to 8 minutes.

Divide the lettuce and cherry tomatoes between two large bowls. To prepare the guacamole, combine the lime juice, avocado oil, salt, scallion, and cilantro in a small bowl. Add the diced avocado and stir to combine, mashing the avocado with a fork if you prefer a smoother consistency. Spoon the meat mixture and guacamole over each bowl of lettuce. Top with salsa and squeeze over additional lime juice and cilantro, if desired.

CLASSIC EGG SALAD

Serves 2

5 large eggs

¼ cup avocado oil mayonnaise

½ scallion, chopped

1 teaspoon Dijon or yellow mustard

1 teaspoon chopped fresh dill

1 teaspoon dill pickle relish (optional)

Salt

Black pepper

Butter lettuce, for serving (optional)

Place the eggs in a saucepan and cover with cold water. Bring the water to a boil and immediately turn off the heat. Cover and let the eggs stand in the hot water for 12 to 15 minutes, then transfer to a bowl of ice water for 5 minutes. Peel and chop the eggs.

In a medium bowl, combine the mayonnaise, scallion, mustard, dill, and pickle relish (if using). Add the eggs and stir to coat evenly with the dressing. Season to taste with salt and pepper and serve in lettuce cups, if desired.

GARDEN SALAD WITH CITRUS DRESSING

Serves 2 to 4

INGREDIENTS

1 carrot

1 yellow squash

½ head lettuce

2 cups spring mix

1 red bell pepper, chopped

½ cup white mushrooms, chopped

For the dressing

2 tablespoons orange juice

2 teaspoons freshly squeezed lime juice

2 teaspoons freshly squeezed lemon juice

6 tablespoons olive oil

½ teaspoon salt

Grate the carrot and slice the squash into thin ribbons using a vegetable peeler. Combine them with the remaining vegetables in a serving bowl. In a small bowl, whisk together the dressing ingredients. Pour the dressing over the salad and toss to combine.

CELERY FENNEL SALAD

Serves 4

INGREDIENTS

1 large fennel bulb

4 celery stalks

3 tablespoons olive oil

2 tablespoons freshly squeezed lemon juice

¼ teaspoon salt

¼ cup fresh basil leaves

Remove the stems and core from the fennel bulb. Slice the fennel as thinly as possible (or use a mandolin). Cut the celery diagonally into thin slices. Combine the fennel and celery with the olive oil, lemon juice, and salt and toss to coat. Stack the basil leaves on top of each other then roll up and slice into thin ribbons. Sprinkle the basil over the salad and serve immediately.

Main Dishes

Vegetarian

BUTTERNUT SQUASH AND LENTIL STEW

Serves 2 to 4

INGREDIENTS

1 tablespoon olive oil

½ onion, diced

2 celery stalks, chopped

1 carrot, diced

1 tablespoon grated fresh ginger

1 pound dry green lentils

½ teaspoon ground cumin

1 teaspoon dried thyme

4 cups low-sodium chicken or vegetable broth

2 cups water

2 teaspoons salt

1 small butternut squash, cubed

In a large pot, heat the oil over medium-high heat and cook the onion, celery, and carrot until the onions are golden, about 5 minutes. Stir in the ginger, lentils, cumin, thyme, broth, water, and salt. Simmer, covered, for 30 minutes. Add the squash, cover, and simmer for an additional 25 minutes, until the squash and lentils are very tender. If using a pressure cooker, combine all the ingredients in the pot and cook at high pressure for 12 minutes. After 5 minutes, release the pressure using the quick release function.

VEGAN PEA PESTO WITH CHICKPEA PASTA

Serves 4

INGREDIENTS

1 teaspoon salt

1 package chickpea or lentil pasta

For the pesto

¼ cup pine nuts or cashews

1 cup frozen peas, thawed

1 small bunch fresh basil

3 garlic cloves, peeled

1 teaspoon salt

1 teaspoon lemon zest

1 tablespoon freshly squeezed lemon juice

¼ cup olive oil

Bring a large pot of water to the boil. Add the salt and pasta and cook according to the package directions.

In a small pan, toast the pine nuts over medium heat until fragrant and slightly brown.

To prepare the pesto, combine the peas, basil, garlic, pine nuts, salt, lemon zest, and lemon juice in a food processor or blender. Pulse until just combined. Add the oil and ¼ cup of cooking water from the pasta. Blend until smooth. Drain the pasta, transfer to a serving dish, and top with the pesto. Toss to combine.

For additional protein, serve with grilled fish or chicken.

BAKED FALAFEL WITH LEMON TAHINI DRESSING

Serves 4

INGREDIENTS

- ⅓ cup olive oil plus **1** tablespoon
- **2** cups cooked chickpeas (or 1 Tetra Pak or 15-ounce can, rinsed and drained)
- **2** teaspoons freshly squeezed lemon juice
- ¼ cup chopped onion
- **2** garlic cloves
- ⅓ cup chopped fresh parsley
- ¼ cup chopped fresh cilantro
- **1** teaspoon ground cumin
- ½ teaspoon salt
- **3** tablespoons gluten-free flour or cornstarch
- ½ teaspoon baking soda

For the dressing

- ¼ cup tahini
- Juice of **1** small lemon
- **1** garlic clove, minced
- **2** tablespoons olive oil
- ½ teaspoon salt
- Black pepper to taste
- ½ cup water
- **1** teaspoon maple syrup (optional)

Preheat the oven to 375°F (190°C). Pour ⅓ cup of olive oil onto a large rimmed baking sheet and tilt to coat evenly.

In a food processor, combine the chickpeas, remaining 1 tablespoon of olive oil, lemon juice, onion, garlic, parsley, cilantro, cumin, and salt. Pulse until combined, leaving the mixture with some texture. Add the flour and baking soda and stir to combine. Take spoonfuls of the mixture and shape into small patties, approximately ½ inch thick. Arrange the patties on the baking sheet and bake for 25 to 30 minutes, flipping after the first 15 minutes.

To prepare the dressing, combine the tahini, lemon juice, garlic, oil, salt, and pepper in a mixing bowl and whisk to combine. Continue whisking while slowly pouring in the water. Alternatively, combine all the ingredients in a blender and blend until smooth. Taste and adjust the proportions if needed, adding more salt, lemon, or tahini. Add the maple syrup, if desired.

PUMPKIN, ARUGULA, AND WHITE BEAN SALAD

Serves 2

INGREDIENTS

1 pound pumpkin or butternut squash, cubed

1 tablespoon olive oil

½ teaspoon salt

1 small package arugula or spring mix

1 cup cooked small white beans, such as great Northern

1 tablespoon pumpkin seeds

For the dressing

Juice of **½** lemon

1 teaspoon maple syrup

2 tablespoons olive oil

½ teaspoon salt

Preheat the oven to 400°F (200°C). Place the pumpkin on a rimmed baking sheet, lightly coat with the olive oil, and sprinkle with the salt. Bake for 25 to 30 minutes, until tender and starting to brown. To prepare the dressing, whisk together the lemon juice, maple syrup, olive oil, and salt. Divide the arugula, white beans, and roasted pumpkin between two bowls. Pour the dressing on top and toss to combine. Top with the pumpkin seeds.

CHICKPEA RATATOUILLE

Serves 2

INGREDIENTS

- **1** onion, chopped
- **1** eggplant, chopped
- **3** tablespoons olive oil
- **1** zucchini, chopped
- **1** yellow (summer) squash
- **1** red bell pepper, chopped
- **2** garlic cloves, minced
- **3** tomatoes, chopped
- **1½** cups cooked chickpeas
- **1** cup cooked lentils
- **1** cup tomato pasta sauce
- **1** tablespoon vinegar
- **½** teaspoon salt
- **½** teaspoon black pepper
- **6** basil leaves, sliced

In a large pan over medium-high heat, cook the onion and eggplant in the olive oil for 5 minutes. Add the remaining ingredients and stir to combine. Cover and simmer for 10 to 15 minutes, stirring occasionally and adding water if needed. (If you prefer vegetables with a firmer texture, add the zucchini, yellow squash, and bell pepper in the final 5 to 10 minutes of cooking.)

Seafood

HONEY-GINGER BROILED SALMON

Serves 2

INGREDIENTS

1 teaspoon grated peeled fresh ginger

½ teaspoon garlic powder

2 tablespoons gluten-free soy sauce

2 tablespoons orange juice

1 tablespoon honey

1 scallion, finely chopped

2 (6-ounce) salmon fillets

In a glass dish approximately the size of the salmon fillets, combine the ginger, garlic powder, soy sauce, orange juice, honey, and scallion. Stir to combine. Add the salmon to the dish, spooning some of the sauce over the top. Refrigerate for 15 to 30 minutes.

Preheat the broiler with the oven rack positioned 4 to 6 inches from the heat source. Line a rimmed baking sheet with foil.

Transfer the salmon to the baking sheet, skin-side down. Broil the salmon for 6 to 10 minutes, until just cooked through.

ASIAN WHOLE FISH WITH BOK CHOY

Serves 2

INGREDIENTS

1 to **2** whole fish, such as snapper, branzino, striped bass

1 lemon, sliced

2 pieces sliced fresh ginger

4 heads baby bok choy

2 garlic cloves, minced

1 teaspoon grated fresh ginger

1 tablespoon olive oil

1 red chili pepper, finely sliced (optional)

¼ cup water

1 tablespoon gluten-free soy sauce

1 teaspoon sugar

2 teaspoons sesame oil

Preheat the oven to 400°F (200°C). Place the fish on a rimmed baking sheet and fill the cavity with the lemon and ginger slices. Bake for 20 to 30 minutes, until the fish flakes easily with a fork.

While the fish is cooking, cut the bok choy into quarters through the stem. In a small pan, cook the garlic, ginger, and chili pepper (if using) in the oil over low heat until fragrant. Add the water, soy sauce, and bok choy. Cover and steam for 3 to 5 minutes. Add the sugar and sesame oil. Stir to combine.

Transfer the fish and bok choy to a plate, pouring over the ginger-garlic sauce.

SHRIMP PAD THAI WITH SHIRATAKI NOODLES

Serves 2

INGREDIENTS

1 package shirataki (konjac) noodles, such as Miracle Noodle Fettuccini*

2 tablespoons avocado, safflower, or light olive oil

3 scallions, sliced

1 red bell pepper, finely sliced

2 garlic cloves, minced

1 cup bean sprouts

1 pound shrimp, peeled and deveined

2 large eggs

For the pad thai sauce

1 tablespoon tamarind paste

1 tablespoon soy sauce or coconut aminos

2 tablespoons fish sauce

2 tablespoons sugar or erythritol

2 tablespoons lime juice or rice vinegar

2 to **3** tablespoons cashew, almond, or peanut butter

1 teaspoon hot sauce

Combine the sauce ingredients and set aside (or use store-bought pad thai sauce).

Drain and rinse the noodles in a colander under running water. Use a knife or kitchen shears to cut to shorter lengths if desired, then place the noodles in a bowl and cover with boiling water for 2 minutes. Drain the noodles again and dry in an unoiled sauté pan over medium-to-low heat for 5 to 10 minutes, until the noodles become opaque and the pan stays dry. Transfer the noodles to a bowl.

 Pour the oil into the pan and add the scallions, bell pepper, garlic, and bean sprouts. Stir fry for 2 minutes. Add the shrimp and cook until pink and opaque, 1 to 2 minutes per side. Push the ingredients to the side to make space in the pan for the eggs. Add slightly more oil if needed and crack the eggs into the pan. Stir the eggs while cooking to break them into small pieces. When the eggs are almost cooked, add the noodles and sauce, stirring to combine. Squeeze over additional lime juice before serving if desired.

* As a substitute for the shirataki noodles, this recipe can also be made with shredded cabbage, spiralized zucchini, spaghetti squash, or a small portion of rice noodles.

NEW ENGLAND BAKED COD

Serves 2

INGREDIENTS

- ½ cup gluten-free breadcrumbs
- 3 tablespoons avocado, safflower, or light olive oil, plus more for greasing baking sheet
- ½ teaspoon onion powder
- ¼ teaspoon salt
- 2 portions cod, haddock, or other white fish

Preheat the oven to 400°F (200°C). Lightly grease a rimmed baking sheet with oil. Combine the breadcrumbs, oil, onion powder, and salt in a bowl. (For additional flavor, add parsley, garlic, dill, lemon pepper, or Old Bay seasoning.) Place the fish on the baking sheet and top with the bread crumb mixture. Bake for 10 to 15 minutes, until the fish is just cooked through.

ROASTED LEMON-GARLIC SHRIMP

Serves 2

INGREDIENTS

1 garlic clove, minced

2 tablespoons olive oil

½ tablespoon chopped fresh parsley

½ teaspoon lemon zest

½ teaspoon salt

1 pound large shrimp, peeled and deveined

1 tablespoon freshly squeezed lemon juice

Preheat the oven to 400°F (200°C). Place the garlic and olive oil in a small glass bowl and microwave for 30 seconds. Add the parsley, lemon zest, and salt to the garlic and oil. Place the shrimp in a pile on a rimmed baking sheet and pour the lemon-garlic mixture on top. Toss the shrimp to coat evenly with the marinade and then arrange in a single layer. Roast for 6 to 8 minutes, until just pink and firm. Sprinkle with the lemon juice before serving.

ASIAN SALT AND PEPPER SHRIMP WITH SNAP PEAS

Serves 2

INGREDIENTS

1 small package sugar snap peas

1 pound shrimp, peeled and deveined

1 teaspoon salt

½ teaspoon Chinese five spice powder

½ teaspoon white pepper

½ teaspoon red pepper flakes, or 1 small fresh red chili pepper (optional)

2 tablespoons avocado or safflower oil

To remove the strings from the sugar snap peas, snap off the tips by hand and pull the string along the length of the pod. In a small bowl, combine the shrimp with the salt, five spice powder, white pepper, and red pepper flakes (if using). Heat the oil in a large fry pan or wok over high heat. Add the sugar snap peas and stir-fry for 2 minutes. Add the shrimp and cook until just opaque in the center.

GREEK SALMON

Serves 2

INGREDIENTS

1 lemon

2 (6-ounce) salmon fillets

½ teaspoon salt

1 tablespoon chopped fresh dill

½ teaspoon dried oregano

½ cup chopped tomatoes

1 shallot, finely chopped

¼ cup Kalamata olives, pitted and halved

Preheat the oven to 425°F (220°C). Cut most of the lemon into ½-inch-thick slices and arrange in a single layer in a baking dish, reserving one end of the lemon to squeeze over the salmon. Place the salmon, skin-side down, on top of the lemon slices. Season with the salt, dill, and oregano and then top with the tomatoes, shallot, and olives. Bake until the salmon is opaque and flakes easily, 12 to 15 minutes. Squeeze lemon juice on top before serving.

MAHI-MAHI WITH SPICY MANGO SALSA

Serves 2

INGREDIENTS

2 (4- to 6-ounce) mahi-mahi fillets

½ teaspoon salt

¼ teaspoon black pepper

1 tablespoon olive oil

For the mango salsa

½ ripe mango, cubed

½ red bell pepper, finely chopped

¼ red onion, chopped

1 tablespoon chopped fresh cilantro

Juice of ½ lime

¼ teaspoon ground ginger

¼ teaspoon ground cumin

¼ teaspoon garlic powder

½ tablespoon pickled jalapeno peppers (optional)

To prepare the mango salsa, combine all the ingredients in a bowl. Set aside.

Dry the surface of the fish fillets with paper towels. Sprinkle with the salt and pepper then grill or pan-fry in the oil over high heat until the fish flakes easily with a fork, 3 to 4 minutes per side. Serve with the mango salsa.

SALMON KATSU

Serves 2

INGREDIENTS

2 (4- to 6-ounce) salmon fillets

1 egg

2 tablespoons cornstarch or gluten-free flour

¼ teaspoon salt

½ teaspoon onion powder

3 tablespoons avocado, safflower, or light olive oil

1 cup gluten-free breadcrumbs (preferably panko)

Remove the skin from the salmon. Cut each fillet into 6 equal pieces, about ½ inch thick. Pat dry with paper towels. Beat the egg in a small bowl. Spread out the breadcrumbs in a separate shallow bowl or plate (alternatively, use crushed rice crackers or Rice Chex cereal).

Combine the cornstarch, salt, and onion powder in a small zip-top bag. Add the salmon pieces and shake to coat evenly.

Heat the oil in a nonstick pan over medium-high heat. Dip each piece of salmon in the egg and then transfer to the bowl with the breadcrumbs. Press the breadcrumbs into the salmon to ensure each piece is evenly coated. Pan-fry for 3 minutes per side or until golden brown and crispy.

WHOLE SNAPPER WITH THAI BASIL AND GINGER SAUCE

Serves 2

INGREDIENTS

1 whole snapper (about 2 pounds)

5 to **10** basil leaves, preferably Thai basil

2 to **3** tablespoons avocado, safflower, or light olive oil

2 tomatoes, chopped

1 red bell pepper, sliced

1 teaspoon grated ginger

2 garlic cloves, minced

1 tablespoon fish sauce

1 tablespoon rice vinegar or lime juice

1 tablespoon sugar or monk fruit/erythritol (optional)

1 teaspoon hot sauce (optional)

1 teaspoon cornstarch (optional)

Preheat the oven to 400°F (200°C). Place the fish on a rimmed baking sheet and stuff with half the basil leaves. Cook until the fish is firm and flakes easily, approximately 30 minutes. While the fish is cooking, prepare the sauce. Heat the oil in a pan over medium-high heat. Add the tomatoes, bell pepper, and ginger and sauté for several minutes. Add the remaining ingredients, lower the heat, and cook for 5 minutes, until the ingredients are well combined. If needed, add 1 to 2 tablespoons of water to thin the sauce or 1 teaspoon of cornstarch to thicken it. Pour the sauce over the fish before serving.

PAN-FRIED SNAPPER FILLETS WITH SALSA VERDE

Serves 2

INGREDIENTS

2 (6-ounce) fish fillets, such as snapper, haddock, or cod

1 tablespoon avocado oil

¼ teaspoon salt

For the salsa verde

½ cup basil leaves

¼ cup mint leaves

¼ cup parsley leaves

½ cup olive oil

1 teaspoon Dijon mustard

1 tablespoon capers

Zest and juice of **½** lemon

1 garlic clove, roughly chopped

To make the salsa verde, combine all the ingredients in a food processor or blender and process until almost smooth. If using fish with skin, score the skin with 3 or 4 diagonal cuts to prevent the fish curling in the pan. Dry the fish with paper towels, coat with the oil, and sprinkle with the salt. Heat a nonstick pan over medium-high heat. Add the fish and cook for 3 to 4 minutes per side. Serve topped with the salsa verde. Leftover salsa verde can be poured over roast or grilled vegetables and keeps refrigerated for several days.

SIMPLE CRISPY-SKIN SALMON WITH TARTAR SAUCE

Serves 2

INGREDIENTS

2 (6-ounce) salmon fillets

1 tablespoon olive oil

Salt

For the tartar sauce

2 teaspoons finely chopped fresh chives

2 teaspoons finely chopped fresh dill

2 teaspoons finely chopped fresh parsley

2 scallions, finely chopped

1 teaspoon capers

4 tablespoons mayonnaise

¼ teaspoon Dijon mustard

Juice of **½** lemon

To prepare the tartar sauce, combine all the ingredients in a bowl. Allow the flavors to meld before serving, preferably for at least 1 hour. Store in the refrigerator for up to 2 days.

Heat a pan over medium heat. Dry the salmon with paper towels and coat with the olive oil and a sprinkle of salt. Place the salmon skin-side down in the pan and continuously push down on the fillets with a spatula for a few minutes to keep the skin in contact with the pan. (Or weigh them down using a metal pot lid smaller than the skillet.) After the first few minutes, push down occasionally until the skin is browned and crispy, about 6 minutes. Flip the salmon to flesh-side down and cook for another 1 to 2 minutes.

CUBAN SALMON

Serves 4

INGREDIENTS

4 (6-ounce) salmon fillets

Zest and juice of **1** lime

1 teaspoon orange zest

¼ cup orange juice

¼ cup finely chopped fresh cilantro

½ tablespoon finely chopped fresh rosemary

¼ cup olive oil

½ teaspoon turmeric

½ teaspoon salt

Remove the skin from the salmon. To prepare the marinade, combine the lime and orange zest and juice, cilantro, rosemary, oil, turmeric, and salt. Add the salmon and marinate for 2 to 6 hours. Remove from the refrigerator 30 minutes before cooking. Pat the salmon dry, then grill, broil, or pan-fry until cooked through.

PARISIAN FISH

Serves 4

INGREDIENTS

3 shallots, finely chopped

2 teaspoons capers, drained

3 tablespoons mayonnaise

1 tablespoon Dijon mustard

1 tablespoon olive oil

1 tablespoon freshly squeezed lemon juice

1 teaspoon grated lemon zest

4 (6-ounce) fish fillets (any flaky white fish)

Chives or parsley, finely chopped, for garnish

Preheat the oven to 425°F (220°C). In a small bowl, combine the shallots, capers, mayonnaise, mustard, olive oil, lemon juice, and lemon zest. Place the fish fillets skin-side down in a shallow baking dish (or remove the skin before cooking). Spread the sauce over the top of each fillet and then bake for 10 to 12 minutes or until the fish flakes easily with a fork. Serve garnished with chives or parsley.

GINGER-LIME FISH PARCELS

Serves 2

INGREDIENTS

2 (6-ounce) fish portions (salmon or any flaky white fish)

1 tablespoon olive oil

Zest and juice of **1** lime

1 (2-inch) piece fresh ginger, thinly sliced

1 scallion, sliced

½ teaspoon salt

Preheat the oven to 400°F. Place each piece of fish on a large square of parchment paper. Brush the fish lightly with the oil, then top each piece with half the lime zest, ginger, scallion, and salt. Bring the edges of the parchment paper together and fold over several times to close into parcels. Bake for 12 to 16 minutes, depending on the thickness of the fish. When cooked through, remove the fish from the parcels, discard the ginger pieces, and sprinkle with the lime juice.

PERUVIAN CEVICHE

Serves 2 to 4

INGREDIENTS

1 pound very fresh white fish (such as halibut), skin removed

½ cup freshly squeezed lime juice

2 scallions (green part only), finely sliced

1 tablespoon chopped fresh cilantro or parsley

1 teaspoon salt

Using a large, very sharp knife, slice the fish into 1½-inch cubes. Place the cubes in a bowl of chilled water. Drain the fish and combine with the lime juice, scallions, cilantro, and salt. Cover and refrigerate for 30 minutes before serving.

PAN-FRIED FISH WITH GREEK HERB SAUCE

Serves 2

INGREDIENTS

1 garlic clove

½ cup plus 1 tablespoon olive oil

¼ cup chopped fresh oregano

¼ cup chopped fresh parsley

2 to **3** tablespoons freshly squeezed lemon juice

½ teaspoon salt

2 fillets flaky white fish, such as snapper or haddock

To prepare the sauce, mince the garlic and add to ½ cup of olive oil in a small pan. Heat gently for 5 minutes (or microwave for 30 to 45 seconds). Blend the garlic and oil with the oregano, parsley, lemon juice, and salt in a blender or small food processor.

When ready to cook the fish, heat the remaining tablespoon of olive oil in a large pan over medium-high heat. Dry the surface of the fish with paper towels and place in the pan, skin-side down. Cook until the skin is crisp and releases from the pan, 3 to 4 minutes. Flip the fish and finish cooking for 1 to 2 minutes longer. Serve with the herb sauce.

SARDINE SALAD

Serves 1

INGREDIENTS

1 can sardines in water

1 scallion, finely chopped

2 tablespoons chopped fresh parsley and/or chives

2 tablespoons freshly squeezed lemon juice

1 tablespoon olive oil

1 teaspoon capers

Bib lettuce or crackers, for serving

Drain and lightly mash the sardines. Combine the sardines with the remaining ingredients and serve in lettuce cups or with crackers.

SHRIMP CAULIFLOWER FRIED RICE

Serves 2

INGREDIENTS

12 ounces cauliflower rice, fresh or frozen

1 pound raw shrimp, peeled and deveined

1 teaspoon salt

2 tablespoons avocado, safflower, or olive oil, divided

2 carrots, peeled and finely diced

½ cup frozen peas, thawed

3 scallions, chopped

2 teaspoons grated fresh ginger

3 garlic cloves, minced

2 large eggs, beaten

2 tablespoons soy sauce or coconut aminos

1 tablespoon sesame oil

1 teaspoon chili sauce or sriracha (optional)

If using frozen cauliflower rice, allow to thaw then drain. If using a whole cauliflower, chop into florets then pulse in a food processor. Season the shrimp with the salt and cook in a large skillet for 1 to 2 minutes per side in 1 tablespoon of oil, until no longer translucent in the center. Transfer the shrimp to a plate.

Lower the heat to medium and add additional oil to the pan if needed. Stir-fry the carrots for 2 to 3 minutes, until they begin to soften. Add the peas, scallions, ginger, garlic, and cauliflower rice and stir-fry until the cauliflower is cooked through. Move the vegetables to the side to create space in the pan and add additional oil if needed.

Crack the eggs into the pan and stir lightly to scramble the eggs while cooking. When the eggs are almost cooked, stir everything to combine. Return the shrimp to the pan and briefly heat through. Add the sesame oil, chili sauce (if using), and additional salt to taste.

Chicken

MOJO CHICKEN

Serves 3 to 4

2 large boneless skinless chicken breasts

Juice of **1** lime

Juice of **½** orange

1 garlic clove, minced

2 tablespoons chopped fresh cilantro

2 teaspoons dried oregano

1 teaspoon dried thyme

1 teaspoon salt

Pound the chicken breasts to an even thickness. In a glass bowl or container large enough to hold the chicken, combine the remaining ingredients. Add the chicken to the marinade, turning to coat it evenly. Refrigerate for at least 1 hour. Preheat the broiler. Transfer the chicken to a foil-lined rimmed baking sheet. Broil under high heat for 5 minutes, then turn off the heat and allow the chicken to stand in the closed oven for an additional 5 to 10 minutes, depending on the thickness of the chicken.

CHICKEN EGG ROLL IN A BOWL

Serves 2

INGREDIENTS

4 to **6** boneless chicken thighs

1 teaspoon salt

½ teaspoon black pepper

2 tablespoons avocado, safflower, or olive oil

1 package coleslaw or broccoli slaw mix, or shredded cabbage and carrots

3 garlic cloves, minced

1 teaspoon peeled and grated fresh ginger

1 to **2** tablespoons soy sauce or coconut aminos

3 scallions, finely chopped, separating white and green parts

1 tablespoon sesame oil

2 teaspoons rice wine vinegar

1 teaspoon hot sauce (optional)

Sprinkle the salt and pepper evenly over the chicken thighs. Heat 1 tablespoon of oil in a large skillet over medium-high heat. Pan-fry the chicken until lightly browned and cooked through, 3 to 5 minutes per side. Transfer the chicken to a cutting board.

Add the remaining 1 tablespoon of oil to the pan, along with the coleslaw mix, garlic, ginger, soy sauce, and the white parts of the scallions. Stir-fry until the vegetables are slightly tender.

Slice the chicken and return it to the pan, along with the green parts of the scallions, sesame oil, vinegar, and hot sauce (if using). Stir-fry briefly until the chicken is heated through.

ONE-PAN MOROCCAN CHICKEN THIGHS WITH CHICKPEAS

Serves 4

INGREDIENTS

1 tablespoon olive oil

8 bone-in chicken thighs

1½ cups cooked chickpeas

½ onion, finely chopped

2 carrots, peeled and chopped

1 red bell pepper, chopped

1 zucchini, chopped

2 garlic cloves, minced

1 teaspoon salt

½ teaspoon black pepper

2 teaspoons ground cumin

2 teaspoons paprika

1 teaspoon ground turmeric

½ teaspoon ground cinnamon

½ teaspoon ground ginger

½ cup chicken broth or water

Juice and zest of **½** lemon

Preheat the oven to 375°F (190°C). Heat the oil in a large, oven-safe skillet over medium-high heat. To start browning the chicken, cook it skin-side down for 5 minutes. Turn the chicken over then add the remaining ingredients, scooping some of the liquid over the chicken. Transfer the pan to the oven and roast until the chicken thighs are cooked through, about 30 minutes.

CHIPOTLE CHICKEN QUINOA BOWLS

Serves 2

INGREDIENTS

2 chicken breast cutlets

1 tablespoon avocado, safflower, or olive oil

2 cups spring greens or chopped romaine lettuce

1 tomato, diced

1 avocado, diced

For the quinoa

1 cup water

½ cup quinoa

½ teaspoon salt

Zest of **1** lime

½ cup chopped fresh cilantro

For the dressing

2 tablespoons olive oil

Juice of **1** lime

1 tablespoon chipotle hot sauce

½ teaspoon salt

1 tablespoon vinegar

To make the quinoa, in a small pot, bring the water to the boil. Add the quinoa and salt. Lower the heat and simmer, covered, until the water is absorbed and the quinoa is tender, about 15 minutes. Remove from the heat and stir in the lime zest and cilantro.

To prepare the dressing, whisk together all the ingredients.

Pan-fry the chicken in the oil until cooked through, about 4 minutes per side. Transfer the chicken to a cutting board and cut into bite-size pieces. Arrange the lettuce, tomato, and avocado in two bowls. Pour over some of the dressing and toss to combine. Add the quinoa and chicken and drizzle with the remaining dressing.

JAMAICAN JERK CHICKEN WITH COCONUT CAULIFLOWER RICE AND BEANS

Serves 2 to 4

INGREDIENTS

1 scallion

1 scotch bonnet or jalapeno pepper, seeds removed

2 garlic cloves

1 teaspoon Chinese five spice powder or ¼ teaspoon allspice

1 teaspoon dried thyme

1 teaspoon chopped fresh ginger

2 tablespoons gluten-free soy sauce or coconut aminos

1 teaspoon avocado oil

4 to **6** boneless skinless chicken thighs

For the coconut rice and beans

1 package riced cauliflower or **½** large cauliflower

2 tablespoons avocado, safflower, or olive oil

1 cup cooked black beans or black-eyed peas

¼ teaspoon salt

¼ cup coconut milk

1 tablespoon chopped fresh cilantro

In a food processor, combine the scallion, chili pepper, garlic, five spice powder, thyme, ginger, soy sauce, and oil. Process until smooth. Pour the sauce over the chicken and marinate, covered, in the refrigerator for at least 2 hours.

If using frozen cauliflower rice, allow to thaw, then drain. If using a whole cauliflower, cut it into florets and then pulse in a food processor to form rice-size pieces. Heat the oil in a large pan over medium heat. Add the cauliflower rice, beans, and salt and cook for 5 minutes, stirring occasionally. Add the coconut milk and cilantro and stir to combine.

Grill or pan-fry the chicken over medium-high heat until cooked through, 4 to 5 minutes per side. Serve with the cauliflower rice and beans.

DAIRY-FREE CHICKEN ALFREDO WITH CHICKPEA PASTA

Serves 2

INGREDIENTS

1 head cauliflower

8 large garlic cloves

2 teaspoons salt

½ box chickpea or lentil pasta

2 chicken breast cutlets, or 1 chicken breast, cut into two thinner layers

3 tablespoons olive oil, divided

½ cup nondairy milk or low-sodium chicken broth

½ teaspoon black pepper

Combine the cauliflower florets, garlic, and salt in a pot and cover with water. Bring to a boil and cook, covered, for 10 minutes or until the cauliflower is very tender.

Meanwhile, cook the pasta according to the package directions. Pan-fry the chicken in 1 tablespoon of olive oil until cooked through, approximately 3 minutes per side.

Drain the cauliflower and garlic and transfer to a blender or food processor. Add the nondairy milk, remaining 2 tablespoons of olive oil, and pepper to the blender and blend for several minutes until smooth, adding additional water or salt if needed. (If your blender container is plastic, it is best to cook the cauliflower in advance and allow it to cool first.)

Slice the chicken into strips. Reheat the sauce if needed and pour the desired amount over the drained pasta and chicken. Extra sauce can be kept for several days in the refrigerator.

CHICKEN AND VEGETABLE SOUP

Serves 8

INGREDIENTS

3 to **4** pounds bone-in chicken pieces or 1 whole chicken, cut into pieces

4 large carrots, divided

4 celery stalks, divided

1 medium onion, cut into quarters

2 teaspoons salt

2 teaspoons dried thyme or 2 fresh sprigs

1 teaspoon dried sage or 5 fresh leaves

2 bay leaves

2 zucchini

½ cup broccoli florets

2 tablespoons chopped fresh parsley

2 tablespoons chopped fresh dill

Place the chicken in a large soup pot and cover with water. Cut 2 carrots and 2 celery sticks into quarters. Add to the pot, along with the onion, salt, thyme, sage, and bay leaves. Simmer for approximately 1½ hours, occasionally skimming the foam that appears on the surface. Use tongs to transfer the chicken pieces to a plate to cool. Use tongs to remove the vegetables and bay leaf and discard (or strain the broth into another pot, discarding the vegetables). Dice the remaining carrots and celery, zucchini, and broccoli, then add them to the broth. Meanwhile, pull the chicken meat from the bones and chop it into small pieces. Return the chicken to the pot, along with the parsley and dill.

CHINESE CHICKEN LETTUCE WRAPS

Serves 2

INGREDIENTS

1 head butter lettuce

3 tablespoons avocado, safflower, or olive oil

1 pound ground chicken

½ medium white onion, finely chopped

2 garlic cloves, minced

2 teaspoons freshly grated ginger or ¼ teaspoon ground ginger

½ cup white mushrooms, finely chopped

2 scallions, chopped

½ teaspoon salt

3 tablespoons soy sauce or coconut aminos

1 tablespoon sesame oil

1 tablespoon almond, cashew, or sunflower butter

2 teaspoons vinegar

1 to **2** teaspoons sugar, erythritol, or sweetener of choice

Separate and rinse the lettuce leaves. Set aside. Heat the oil in a large pan over medium-high heat. Add the chicken, onion, garlic, ginger, and mushrooms. Cook over high heat for 5 to 8 minutes, breaking up the chicken. Add the scallions, salt, soy sauce, sesame oil, almond butter, vinegar, and sugar. Cook for 2 to 3 minutes more and adjust the seasoning if needed. Serve in lettuce cups.

GRILLED ITALIAN LEMON CHICKEN

Serves 2

INGREDIENTS

2 boneless skinless chicken breasts

3 tablespoons olive oil

2 tablespoons freshly squeezed lemon juice

1 tablespoon finely chopped fresh rosemary

2 garlic cloves, sliced

1 teaspoon grated lemon zest

Pound the chicken breasts to an even thickness then transfer to a glass bowl or baking dish. Add the remaining ingredients and marinate for 30 minutes at room temperature or several hours refrigerated. Grill or pan-fry the chicken until cooked through, 3 to 5 minutes on each side.

LEMON-HERB ROAST CHICKEN WITH CARROTS AND BRUSSELS SPROUTS

Serves 4

INGREDIENTS

1 lemon, zested then quartered

1 tablespoon fresh thyme or 2 teaspoons dried

1 teaspoon dried sage or dried mixed herbs

4 tablespoons olive oil, divided

2 teaspoons salt, divided

1 whole (4- to 5-pound) chicken

6 garlic cloves

3 large carrots, chopped

1 pound Brussels sprouts, halved

Preheat the oven to 425°F (220°C). To prepare the herb rub, combine the lemon zest in a small bowl with the thyme, sage, 2 tablespoons of olive oil and 1 teaspoon of salt. Remove any giblets from the chicken cavity and dry the outside with paper towels. Gently separate the skin from the chicken breasts and add spoonfuls of the herb rub to the space underneath the skin. Cover with the skin again and rub the outside to evenly distribute the herb mixture. Rub any leftover mixture (or a drizzle of olive oil and salt) over the outside of the bird.

Stuff the chicken cavity with the lemon quarters and whole garlic cloves. Roast for 1 hour, 15 minutes until the juices run clear when a knife is inserted near the thigh.

While the chicken is cooking, arrange the carrots and Brussels sprouts on a rimmed baking sheet and coat with the remaining 2 tablespoons of olive oil and 1 teaspoon of salt. Transfer to the oven after the first 45 minutes of cooking time. Allow the chicken to rest for 5 to 10 minutes before serving.

CHICKEN SOUVLAKI WITH AVOCADO TZATZIKI

Serves 4

INGREDIENTS

2 garlic cloves, sliced

¼ cup chopped fresh oregano or 2 tablespoons dried

1 teaspoon dried marjoram, rosemary, or mixed herbs

¼ cup olive oil

Zest and juice of **½** lemon (2 to 3 tablespoons)

1 teaspoon sea salt

2 large boneless skinless chicken breasts

For the avocado tzatziki

1 avocado

1 cucumber, grated

1 tablespoon garlic-infused oil

Juice of **½** lemon

½ teaspoon salt

1 tablespoon chopped fresh dill

In a small microwave-safe bowl, combine the garlic, oregano, marjoram, and olive oil. Microwave for 45 seconds. Pour the mixture into a large glass bowl or container, reserving 1 tablespoon for the tzatziki sauce. Add the lemon zest, lemon juice, and salt, and whisk to combine.

To ensure the chicken cooks evenly without drying out, place in a large zip-top bag and pound to an equal thickness, or cut each chicken breast in half to form thinner cutlets. Add the chicken breasts to the marinade and allow to sit for 30 minutes at room temperature. Grill or pan-fry the chicken until cooked through, 4 to 5 minutes per side.

To prepare the avocado tzatziki, mash the avocado and combine with the remaining ingredients.

CHICKEN FLORENTINE

Serves 2

INGREDIENTS

2 boneless skinless chicken breasts

1 teaspoon dried thyme or Italian seasoning

½ teaspoon salt, plus more

4 tablespoons olive oil, divided

1 (8-ounce) package small mushrooms, quartered

2 garlic cloves, minced

1 shallot, minced

1 (6- to 8-ounce) package baby spinach

Pound the chicken to an even thickness. Sprinkle the chicken with the thyme and salt. Set a cast-iron skillet over medium heat and add 2 tablespoons of olive oil. Add the chicken and cook until lightly brown, about 5 minutes on each side.

Meanwhile, in a separate pan, heat the remaining 2 tablespoons of olive oil over medium heat. Add the mushrooms, garlic, and shallot and sauté for 5 minutes. Add the spinach, then cover the pan and cook until the spinach wilts. Stir well and add salt to taste. To serve, top each chicken breast with the spinach and mushroom mixture.

CHICKEN STIR-FRY WITH GINGER AND GARLIC

Serves 4

INGREDIENTS

8 boneless chicken thighs

3 tablespoons olive oil, divided

1 to **2** cups sliced red cabbage

1 zucchini, sliced

1 cup mushrooms, sliced

2 tablespoons grated ginger

3 garlic cloves, minced

2 scallions (green parts), sliced

1 teaspoon salt

½ teaspoon white pepper

¼ cup water

Pan-fry the chicken thighs in 1 tablespoon of olive oil over high heat, 3 to 5 minutes per side. Meanwhile, in a separate large pan, heat the remaining 2 tablespoons of olive oil over medium heat. Add the cabbage, zucchini, mushrooms, ginger, garlic, scallions, salt, pepper, and water. Cover the pan and steam the vegetables for 5 minutes, then uncover and continue stir-frying until tender. Slice the chicken thighs, then add them to the pan with the vegetables. Toss to combine.

RANCH CHICKEN WRAP

Serves 2

INGREDIENTS

2 tablespoons mayonnaise

1 tablespoon olive oil

1 tablespoon freshly squeezed lemon juice

1 tablespoon chopped fresh dill

1 tablespoon chopped fresh parsley or chives

½ teaspoon onion powder (optional)

½ teaspoon mustard (optional)

½ avocado, mashed

1 scallion, finely chopped

1 celery stalk, finely chopped

2 roast chicken breasts, cubed

Lettuce, collards, or kale for serving

Whisk together the mayonnaise, oil, lemon juice, dill, parsley, onion powder, and mustard. Add the mashed avocado, scallion, and celery, then stir in the chicken. Serve in lettuce cups or wrap in a collard or kale leaf (with the rib removed).

CHICKEN WITH MUSHROOMS AND SAGE (INSTANT POT)

Serves 4

INGREDIENTS

2 tablespoons olive oil

4 garlic cloves, sliced

8 skinless boneless chicken thighs

2 cups mushrooms, halved

8 fresh sage leaves, chopped

½ cup water

½ teaspoon dried thyme

½ teaspoon sea salt

2 tablespoons chopped fresh basil

Set the Instant Pot to sauté. Combine the olive oil and garlic in the pot and lightly brown the chicken thighs. Add the mushrooms, sage, water, thyme, and salt. Close the lid and cook at high pressure for 15 minutes (or 25 minutes if the chicken is frozen). Quick release the pressure. Serve topped with the basil.

Alternate cooking method: Brown the chicken in an oven-safe cast-iron pan. Add the remaining ingredients and braise in a 325°F oven for 30 to 40 minutes.

CHICKEN SINGAPORE NOODLES WITH SPAGHETTI SQUASH

Serves 2 to 3

INGREDIENTS

- **1** medium spaghetti squash
- **4** boneless skinless chicken thighs
- **2** tablespoons avocado, safflower, or light olive oil
- **½** teaspoon salt
- **2** garlic cloves, minced
- **½** onion
- **2** heads baby bok choy
- **1** red bell pepper
- **1** cup snow peas
- **2** teaspoons yellow or madras curry powder
- **2** scallions, finely chopped

To prepare the spaghetti squash, cut it in half and scoop out the seeds. Place it, cut-sides down, in a microwave-safe dish. Add water to a depth of 1 inch and microwave for 20 minutes, until fork tender. Alternatively, steam the squash halves in an Instant Pot for 10 to 15 minutes with quick release, or coat lightly with oil and oven bake for 40 minutes at 425°F (220°C).

While the squash cooks, cut the chicken thighs into bite-size pieces and slice all the vegetables so they are ready when needed. When the squash is cooked, scoop out the strands and set them aside. In a large, deep skillet or wok, fry the chicken in the oil over medium-high heat until it begins to brown, 3 to 5 minutes. Add the salt, garlic, onion, bok choy, bell pepper, and snow peas. Stir-fry until the vegetables are just tender. Add the cooked spaghetti squash, curry powder, and scallions. Stir-fry until the ingredients are well combined.

DAIRY-FREE CREAMY CHICKEN STEW (INSTANT POT)

Serves 4

INGREDIENTS

- **8** skinless boneless chicken thighs
- **1** large leek
- **3** medium carrots, roughly chopped
- **1** medium celeriac (celery root), peeled and roughly chopped
- **¾** cup water
- **1** teaspoon turmeric
- **1** bay leaf
- **1** garlic clove
- **¾** cup frozen peas

Cut each chicken thigh into quarters. Slice the leek into rings and soak in water to remove any sandy residue, rinsing well and then draining. Combine the chicken, leek, carrots, celeriac, water, turmeric, bay leaf, and garlic in the Instant Pot and cook at high pressure for 17 minutes, with 5 minutes natural release. Remove some of the broth, celeriac, and carrots and puree before returning to the pot. Add the frozen peas and allow to stand until the peas are warmed through.

Beef

STEAK WITH ARGENTINIAN CHIMICHURRI

Serves 2

INGREDIENTS

2 (6-ounce) steaks

½ teaspoon salt

¾ cup extra-virgin olive oil, plus **1** tablespoon

2 garlic cloves, sliced

1 bunch flat-leaf parsley

Zest and juice of **1** lemon

1 tablespoon diced onion

Take the steaks out of the refrigerator 30 minutes before cooking and sprinkle with the salt. In a small pan, warm ¾ cup of olive oil with the garlic for 5 minutes (or microwave for 45 seconds). To prepare the chimichurri sauce, process the garlic and oil mixture with the parsley, lemon zest and juice, and onion in a blender or food processor.

To prepare the steaks, preheat the oven to 325°F. Dry the steaks thoroughly with a paper towel then coat with the remaining 1 tablespoon of olive oil. Heat an oven-safe cast-iron pan over medium-high heat. Briefly sear the steaks on one side, 2 to 3 minutes. Flip the steaks and transfer the pan to the oven to finish cooking, about 5 minutes for rare, 10 minutes for well done. (Use caution removing the pan from the oven, as the handle will be hot.) Allow to rest for 5 minutes before serving with the chimichurri.

BURGER SALAD

Serves 4

2 pounds lean ground beef

½ teaspoon salt

1 tablespoon olive oil

For the salad

1 cup mushrooms, sliced

2 radishes, sliced

2 small cucumbers, sliced

1 head lettuce

1 avocado, pitted and sliced

For the dressing

¼ cup olive oil

2 tablespoons Dijon mustard

Juice of **½** lemon

Shape the ground beef into four large patties. Heat a grill pan over medium-high heat. Lightly coat the burger patties with the salt and olive oil. Grill for 3 to 5 minutes on each side until cooked through.

In a small bowl, whisk together the dressing ingredients.

Combine the mushrooms, radishes, cucumbers, and lettuce in a large bowl. Dress the salad and toss to combine. Serve to individual plates and then top with the burger patties and sliced avocado.

BEEF AND CABBAGE STIR-FRY

Serves 4

INGREDIENTS

2 pounds lean ground beef

2 tablespoons olive oil

½ red cabbage, shredded

2 garlic cloves, sliced

½ teaspoon powdered ginger or 1 teaspoon minced fresh

1 teaspoon salt

2 scallions, chopped

3 small bunches baby bok choy, chopped

1 tablespoon freshly squeezed lemon or lime juice

Sauté the ground beef in the olive oil until cooked through, then transfer to a bowl. In the same pan, sauté the cabbage with the garlic, ginger, and salt until the cabbage is tender, approximately 5 minutes. Add the scallions, bok choy, cooked beef, and lemon juice. Cook for 1 to 2 minutes more, then serve.

TURKISH BEEF KEBABS

Serves 4

INGREDIENTS

¼ cup minced fresh parsley

2 teaspoons finely chopped fresh rosemary

1 teaspoon dried oregano

1 scallion, finely chopped

1 teaspoon salt

1 pinch saffron (optional)

2 pounds lean ground beef

In a large mixing bowl, combine all the ingredients. Shape into sausages and place on skewers to grill for 3 to 5 minutes per side, or bake at 425°F (220°C) for 10 to 15 minutes.

KEFTEDES (GREEK MEATBALLS) WITH DAIRY-FREE TZATZIKI

Serves 2 to 3

INGREDIENTS

1 pound lean ground beef

½ zucchini

⅓ onion, grated

1 garlic clove, minced

1 teaspoon salt

½ teaspoon black pepper

2 tablespoons chopped fresh parsley

1 teaspoon dried oregano

¼ teaspoon dried cumin

¼ teaspoon ground cinnamon

2 tablespoons olive oil

For the tzatziki

⅓ seedless cucumber (also known as English or hothouse)

3 tablespoons avocado oil mayonnaise

½ garlic clove, minced

1 tablespoon olive oil

1 tablespoon freshly squeezed lemon juice

1 tablespoon chopped fresh parsley or dill

Salt

Black pepper

Peel and grate the zucchini. Taking small handfuls of the grated zucchini, squeeze out moisture and then transfer to a bowl. Combine the ground beef, zucchini, onion, garlic, salt, pepper, parsley, oregano, cumin, and cinnamon. Mix to combine. Scoop out mixture to form 1½-inch-diameter meatballs. Fry in the olive oil over medium heat for 2 to 3 minutes per side or bake at 425°F (220°C) for 10 to 15 minutes until cooked through.

To prepare the tzatziki, grate the cucumber and transfer to a small bowl. Add the mayonnaise, garlic, olive oil, lemon juice, and parsley. Season to taste with salt and pepper.

Serve the meatballs with the tzatziki sauce for dipping. This dish also pairs well with a Greek salad.

UNSTUFFED CABBAGE ROLLS

Serves 4 to 6

INGREDIENTS

2 pounds lean ground beef

1 tablespoon olive oil

1 large onion, chopped

3 garlic cloves, minced

1 large carrot, grated

1 teaspoon paprika

¾ cup brown lentils

1 (24- to 32-ounce) jar tomato pasta sauce

3 cups water

2 teaspoons salt

½ small head cabbage, chopped

2 tablespoons vinegar

2 tablespoons sugar or erythritol (optional)

In a large pot or deep skillet, lightly brown the beef in the olive oil over medium-high heat for 3 to 5 minutes. Add the onion, garlic, carrot, paprika, lentils, pasta sauce, water, and salt. Bring to the boil, cover, the lower the heat to medium and simmer for 10 minutes, stirring occasionally. Add the cabbage, vinegar, and sweetener (if using). Simmer for 15 minutes or until the cabbage and lentils are tender. If needed, uncover the pot for the final 5 minutes to allow excess liquid to evaporate.

Pork

PORK TENDERLOIN WITH MUSTARD AND THYME

Serves 2 to 4

1 garlic clove, minced

1 tablespoon chopped fresh rosemary

1 tablespoon chopped fresh thyme

2 tablespoons olive oil

1 teaspoon Dijon mustard

1 teaspoon salt

1 (1- to 2 -pound) pork tenderloin

In a small bowl, combine the garlic, rosemary, thyme, olive oil, mustard, and salt. Rub this mixture over the pork tenderloin then refrigerate for at least 2 hours or overnight. Take out of the refrigerator 30 minutes before cooking.

Preheat the oven to 400°F (200°C). Roast for 20 to 25 minutes or until a thermometer shows an internal temperature of 145°F (65°C). (Additional time may be needed if the tenderloin is larger than 1½ pounds.) Rest the pork for 5 minutes before serving.

This recipe can also be made by doubling the quantity of herbs, garlic, and oil, and roasting at 350°F (175°C) for 1 to 1½ hours.

VIETNAMESE PORK TENDERLOIN

Serves 4

INGREDIENTS

1 (3-inch) fresh lemongrass stalk

2 garlic cloves

¼ red onion

2 teaspoons soy sauce or coconut aminos

1 tablespoon fish sauce

1 tablespoon sugar

1 tablespoon avocado oil

1 (1- to 2 -pound) pork tenderloin

To prepare the marinade, place the lemongrass, garlic, and onion in a food processor or blender. Pulse to combine. Add the soy sauce, fish sauce, sugar, and oil. Blend until smooth. Place the pork in a large glass dish. Pour the marinade on top and turn to coat the pork evenly. Cover and refrigerate for at least 1 hour and up to 24 hours.

Preheat the oven to 400°F (200°C). Transfer the pork to a rimmed baking sheet. Roast for 20 to 25 minutes or until a thermometer shows an internal temperature of 145°F (65°C). Rest the pork for 5 minutes before serving.

PORK SCHNITZEL

Serves 2

INGREDIENTS

2 boneless pork loin chops

1 egg

1 cup gluten-free breadcrumbs (preferably panko)

¼ teaspoon paprika

2 tablespoons cornstarch or gluten-free flour

1 teaspoon salt

1 teaspoon garlic powder

¼ teaspoon black pepper

4 tablespoons avocado or sunflower oil

½ lemon, cut into wedges

Trim the fat from the pork chops. If using thick chops, cut in half to form thinner cutlets. Place the pork chops in a large zip-top bag (or between two layers of parchment paper) and pound to a thickness of ¼ inch. Cut several slits around the edges to stop the pork curling during cooking. In a shallow bowl, beat the egg. In a separate shallow bowl, mix together the breadcrumbs and paprika.

Add the cornstarch, salt, garlic powder, and pepper to the zip-top bag and shake to coat the pork evenly (or sprinkle over each side of the pork). Heat the oil in a nonstick pan over medium-high heat. Dip each piece of pork in the egg mixture and then the breadcrumbs, pressing the crumbs to coat the pork evenly. Pan-fry for 2 to 3 minutes per side. Serve with a wedge of lemon.

PORK CHOPS PIZZAIOLA

Serves 2

2 tablespoons olive oil

2 bone-in pork chops

½ medium onion, chopped

1 red bell pepper, sliced

1 garlic clove, minced

1 cup tomato pasta sauce

1 fresh tomato, chopped

1 teaspoon dried oregano

1 teaspoon fennel seeds

½ teaspoon salt

Heat the oil in a pan over medium-high heat. Cook the pork chops for 3 minutes per side, until slightly brown. Transfer to a plate. Add the onion to the same pan and cook for 5 minutes. Add the bell pepper, garlic, pasta sauce, chopped tomato, oregano, fennel seeds, and salt. Simmer for 5 minutes, stirring. Return the pork to the pan and heat through, spooning over the sauce. Thicker pork chops may require an additional 5 minutes to finish cooking in the sauce.

Turkey

TURKEY BURGERS

Serves 4

INGREDIENTS

1 medium zucchini

1 carrot

1½ pounds lean ground turkey

1 teaspoon salt

½ teaspoon onion powder

1 tablespoon avocado, safflower, or olive oil

Grate the zucchini, then wrap in a clean kitchen towel and squeeze out as much moisture as possible. Grate the carrot and combine with the zucchini, turkey, salt, and onion powder. Form the mixture into patties then pan-fry in the oil over medium-high heat for about 4 minutes each side or until cooked through.

TURKEY MEATBALL SOUP

Serves 4

INGREDIENTS

2 carrots

2 celery stalks

3 cups low-sodium chicken broth

1½ pounds lean ground turkey

1 tablespoon olive or avocado oil

1 teaspoon salt

Combine the carrots, celery, and broth in a pot over medium-high heat. While the vegetables begin to cook, prepare the meatballs. Combine the turkey, oil, and salt in a bowl and form into 1-inch meatballs. Add the meatballs to the broth and then simmer over low heat for 10 to 15 minutes or until cooked through.

TURKEY QUINOA MEATLOAF

Serves 4

INGREDIENTS

- **1** cup uncooked white quinoa
- **2** cups water
- **1** onion, roughly chopped
- **1** medium carrot, cut into large chunks
- **1** small package cremini mushrooms, stalks removed
- **¼** cup fresh parsley
- **1** tablespoon olive oil
- **2** garlic cloves, minced
- **1** teaspoon salt
- **½** teaspoon black pepper
- **2** teaspoons Worcestershire sauce
- **¼** cup ketchup or tomato pasta sauce
- **1** egg, beaten
- **1½** pounds ground turkey
- **2** teaspoons lemon zest (optional)

To prepare the quinoa, place it in a fine mesh colander and rinse under running water for several minutes to remove any bitterness. Transfer the quinoa to a saucepan and add the water, bringing it to a boil. Lower the heat and simmer, uncovered, until the water is absorbed, about 15 minutes. Turn off the heat, cover, and allow to stand for 5 minutes.

Preheat the oven to 400°F (200°C). Pulse the onion, carrot, mushrooms, and parsley in a food processor or blender to form small, rice-size pieces. In a large skillet over medium heat, combine the vegetable mixture, oil, garlic, salt, and pepper. Cook for 5 to 10 minutes, until any liquid evaporates and the vegetables are soft. Transfer to a bowl. Add the Worcestershire sauce, ketchup, egg, turkey, and ¾ cup of cooked quinoa. Mix to combine.

Mound the mixture into a loaf shape on a rimmed baking sheet. Top with additional ketchup or tomato sauce, if desired. Bake for 50 minutes or until the center reaches 160°F (70°C). Cover with foil and allow to rest for 10 minutes before slicing. Serve with additional quinoa as a side dish, adding salt and lemon zest to taste.

TURKEY AND LENTIL STUFFED PEPPERS

Serves 4

INGREDIENTS

1 pound ground turkey or lean beef

1 small onion, finely chopped

1 jalapeno pepper

1 teaspoon ground cumin

1 tablespoon olive oil

2 garlic cloves, minced

1 large tomato, diced

2 cups cooked lentils

1 teaspoon salt

4 large red bell peppers

⅓ cup water or chicken broth

½ avocado, chopped

¼ cup chopped fresh cilantro or 1 scallion, finely chopped

In a large pan, sauté the turkey, onion, jalapeno pepper, and cumin in the olive oil over medium-high heat until the turkey is lightly browned. Add the garlic, diced, lentils, and salt, and then simmer for 10 minutes, covered. Meanwhile, cut the bell peppers in half horizontally and remove the white ribs and seeds. Place them cut-side up in a baking dish. Fill the peppers with the lentil and turkey mixture. Pour the water into the baking dish and cover tightly with foil. Bake for 45 minutes. Serve topped with the avocado and cilantro.

Lamb

ROAST LEG OF LAMB

Serves 8 to 10

INGREDIENTS

10 garlic cloves, finely chopped

½ cup fresh rosemary leaves

½ tablespoon salt

¼ cup olive oil

1 (5-pound) boneless leg of lamb, tied with netting

Preheat the oven to 425°F (220°C). In a small bowl, combine the garlic, rosemary, salt, and olive oil. Rub the herb and garlic mixture over the lamb to coat. (If it is tied with stretchy netting, remove the netting, unroll the lamb, and coat the inner surface with the mixture before rolling back up and re-covering with the netting.)

Place the lamb in a roasting pan and transfer to the oven. After 15 minutes, turn the oven down to 325°F (165°C) and continue roasting for another 1½ to 2 hours. Cover tightly with foil and let rest for 20 minutes before carving.

LAMB SHAWARMA SALAD

Serves 2

INGREDIENTS

12 ounces leftover roast lamb

2 tablespoons olive oil

2 teaspoons chopped fresh rosemary or ½ teaspoon dried

1 teaspoon dried oregano

½ teaspoon salt

½ head lettuce

For the tzatziki dressing

1 cucumber, grated

1 avocado, mashed

1 tablespoon olive oil

2 tablespoons freshly squeezed lemon juice

2 teaspoons chopped fresh dill

1 to **2** tablespoons water (if needed)

Combine the ingredients for the tzatziki dressing and set aside. Thinly slice the leftover roast lamb (this is even easier if the lamb is still slightly frozen). Fry the lamb in the olive oil with the rosemary, oregano, and salt, until warmed through and slightly browned. Serve over the lettuce, topped with the tzatziki dressing.

MOROCCAN LAMB STEW (INSTANT POT)

Serves 4

INGREDIENTS

2 pounds lean lamb stew meat

1 tablespoon olive oil

3 carrots, chopped

1½ cups cooked chickpeas

1 (2-inch) piece fresh ginger, grated

1 teaspoon dried rosemary

Zest and juice of 1 orange

1 tablespoon maple syrup

1 teaspoon salt

1 cup water

2 zucchini, chopped

2 tablespoons chopped fresh parsley or cilantro

With the Instant Pot set to sauté, lightly brown the lamb in the olive oil. Add the carrots, chickpeas, ginger, rosemary, orange zest and juice, maple syrup, salt, and water. Close the lid and cook at high pressure for 35 minutes. Manually release the pressure, then add the zucchini and cilantro and set to sauté for 5 minutes until the zucchini softens and the sauce reduces.

(Alternatively, lightly brown the lamb in a large Dutch oven. Add the remaining ingredients then simmer over low heat for 1½ hours, adding the zucchini in the final 5 minutes.)

Side Dishes

LOW-CARB ROSEMARY FLATBREAD

Serves 4 *Recipe inspired by Arman Liew*

INGREDIENTS

12 egg whites

¼ cup coconut flour

1 teaspoon dried rosemary

1 teaspoon dried oregano

½ teaspoon salt

2 teaspoons baking powder

Olive oil

In a large bowl, whisk together the egg whites, coconut flour, rosemary, oregano, salt, and baking powder.

Heat the olive oil in a medium pan with a lid over low heat. Pour one-quarter of the mixture into the pan and cover with the lid. Cook for 2 to 4 minutes or until bubbles appear around the edge of the flatbread. Use a large spatula to flip and cook for an additional 2 minutes. Repeat the process with the remaining mixture to make four flatbreads. The flatbreads can be fragile when warm, so it is best to let them cool before using.

BRUSSELS SPROUT CHIPS

Serves 2 to 4

INGREDIENTS

1 pound large Brussels sprouts

2 tablespoons avocado, safflower, or light olive oil

½ teaspoon salt

Preheat the oven to 325°F (165°C). Cut the end off each Brussels sprout, and then halve. Make a triangular cut at the base of each half to help release the leaves from the inner stalk. Separate the leaves and spread them out on a rimmed baking sheet. (The inner cores will not become crispy but can be roasted on the same baking sheet or reserved for another recipe). Spray or lightly drizzle the sprouts with the oil, tossing to make sure the leaves are evenly coated. Roast for 15 to 20 minutes or until lightly browned and crispy. Sprinkle with the salt before serving.

KALE SLAW

Serves 4

INGREDIENTS

½ head red cabbage

4 large kale leaves

3 carrots

For the dressing

¼ cup olive oil

¼ cup freshly squeezed lemon juice

2 tablespoons finely chopped fresh parsley

1 tablespoon chopped fresh basil

1 scallion, finely chopped

1 teaspoon maple syrup

½ teaspoon salt

Shred the cabbage in a food processor (or finely slice). Remove the ribs from the kale and finely chop the leaves. Grate the carrots. To prepare the dressing, whisk together all the ingredients, then pour the dressing over the vegetables, tossing to coat. Refrigerate for at least 30 minutes before serving.

FENNEL SLAW

Serves 4

1 fennel bulb

½ head cabbage, shredded

2 scallions, finely chopped

For the dressing

2 tablespoons avocado oil mayonnaise

1 tablespoon olive oil

Juice of **½** lemon

1 teaspoon honey, maple syrup, or erythritol

1 teaspoon sea salt

1 tablespoon chopped fresh parsley

2 tablespoons roughly chopped fennel fronds

Quarter the fennel bulb, remove the core, and slice the bulb thinly. Reserve some fennel fronds for the dressing. Combine the sliced fennel with the cabbage and scallions. Combine the dressing ingredients in a small bowl and whisk. Pour the dressing over the vegetables and toss to coat.

KALE CHIPS

Serves 2 to 4

INGREDIENTS

1 bunch kale

1 tablespoon olive oil

½ teaspoon sea salt

Preheat the oven to 275°F. Wash the kale and dry thoroughly using paper towels (or wash well in advance and allow to dry). Remove the center ribs and tear or cut the kale leaves into large pieces. Pile the leaves on a large rimmed baking sheet and lightly coat with the olive oil and salt. Mix with your hands then spread the kale out evenly across the baking sheet. If the leaves are overlapping, it may be necessary to split into two batches or use two trays. Bake until crisp, about 20 minutes.

SAUTÉED KALE

Serves 2 to 4

1 bunch kale

2 garlic cloves, sliced

2 tablespoons olive oil

¼ cup water

½ teaspoon sea salt

Juice of **½** lemon

Remove the center ribs and cut the kale leaves into large pieces. In a deep pan, cook the garlic in the olive oil over medium heat for 2 to 5 minutes. Add the kale, water, and salt. Cover the pan for 3 minutes. Uncover and continue cooking for another few minutes. Squeeze the lemon juice over the kale and serve.

ITALIAN MARINATED VEGETABLES

Serves 4 to 6

INGREDIENTS

- **1** head cauliflower, cut into small florets
- **2** carrots, peeled and sliced
- **1** zucchini, sliced
- **1** pound small mushrooms, stems removed, halved
- **1** cup frozen artichoke hearts, thawed
- **¼** cup olive oil
- **¼** cup vinegar
- **2** tablespoons freshly squeezed lemon juice
- **1** teaspoon salt
- **1** garlic clove, minced
- **4** fresh basil leaves, sliced
- **1** teaspoon dried oregano
- **1** teaspoon dried thyme

Steam or boil the cauliflower florets and carrots for 3 minutes. Add the zucchini and cook an additional 1 to 2 minutes, until slightly tender. Transfer the cooked vegetables to a large bowl and add the mushrooms and artichoke hearts. Whisk together the olive oil, vinegar, lemon juice, salt, garlic, and herbs. Pour the dressing over the vegetables and toss to combine. Allow to marinate for at least 30 minutes. Serve at room temperature.

FRIED CABBAGE WITH HAM

Serves 4 to 6

INGREDIENTS

3 slices ham or Canadian bacon

3 tablespoons olive oil

1 head cabbage, chopped

½ teaspoon salt

¼ cup water

Dice the ham and fry in the olive oil until lightly browned. Add the cabbage, salt, and water. Cover the pan and cook over medium heat for 5 minutes. Remove the lid and continue cooking until the cabbage is tender, stirring and adding additional olive oil if needed.

Desserts

A Note About Sweeteners

When making desserts, it is your choice whether to use conventional sugar, maple syrup, honey, or a sugar alternative such as erythritol or monk fruit.

The small amount of sugar called for in these recipes will have some impact on blood sugar levels, but the impact is lessened by the presence of fat, protein, and fiber from the remaining ingredients. The recipes avoid refined starches, to further reduce blood sugar impact.

If you would prefer to replace some or all of the sugar in a recipe with a sugar alternative, the best option is typically a combination of erythritol and monk fruit extract, which will have a 1:1 conversion to regular sugar and no glycemic impact. Good options include

- Lakanto Monkfruit Sweetener

- Whole Earth Sweetener Co. Monk Fruit with Erythritol

- Swerve Granular Sweetener

Pure erythritol (without added monk fruit or stevia) will typically have 70 percent of the sweetness of sugar, so you may need to add more to taste.

A Note about Using Beans for Dessert Recipes

Several recipes in this chapter use beans in place of refined flours, to increase protein and fiber and keep blood sugar levels steady. For optimal results, it is best to soak beans overnight and cook until soft, ideally in a pressure cooker. Using canned beans will produce a stronger bean flavor and heavier texture. This can be minimized to some extent by rinsing the beans very well and boiling for an additional 5 to 10 minutes before use in a recipe.

You can typically substitute any bean for the specific type called for in a recipe, but black-eyed peas, chickpeas, adzuki beans, and great Northern beans typically produce the best results.

WALNUT FUDGE BROWNIES

Serves 16 *Recipe inspired by Christina Curp*

1 cup unsweetened cocoa powder

1½ cups cooked butternut squash or pumpkin

4 large eggs

⅔ cup sugar, maple syrup, or erythritol

⅔ cup avocado or safflower oil

⅓ cup cashew, almond, or sunflower seed butter

2 teaspoons baking powder

½ teaspoon salt

2 teaspoons pure vanilla extract

¾ cup walnuts, chopped

Preheat the oven to 350°F (175°C). Grease an 8-inch square baking pan.

Combine all the ingredients, except for the walnuts, in a blender or food processor and blend until smooth. Stir in the walnuts. Pour the batter into the baking pan. Bake for 40 minutes or until the center is firm to the touch. Allow to cool for 20 minutes before cutting.

PECAN CHOCOLATE CHIP BLONDIES

Serves 16

INGREDIENTS

1½ cups cooked white beans or chickpeas

½ cup rolled oats

2 tablespoons avocado or safflower oil

2 tablespoons peanut, cashew, or sunflower seed butter

⅓ cup maple syrup or erythritol

½ teaspoon baking powder

½ teaspoon baking soda

¼ teaspoon salt

2 teaspoons pure vanilla extract

⅓ cup dark chocolate chips

½ cup chopped pecans

Preheat the oven to 350°F (175°C). Grease an 8-inch square baking pan.

Combine all the ingredients except the chocolate chips and pecans in a food processor and process until smooth. Stir in the chocolate chips and half the pecans. Pour the batter into the baking pan. Top with the remaining pecans, pressing them into the batter lightly with the back of a spoon. Bake for 20 minutes or until golden brown and firm in the center. Allow to cool in the pan for 15 minutes before cutting.

FLOURLESS PEANUT BUTTER COOKIES

Makes 20 cookies

INGREDIENTS

1 cup peanut butter

½ cup brown sugar

¼ cup erythritol

1 teaspoon pure vanilla extract

1 egg

1 teaspoon baking powder

Preheat the oven to 350°F (175°C). Using an electric mixer, beat together the peanut butter, sugar, erythritol, and vanilla. Add the egg and baking powder and mix until smooth. Using a tablespoon measure, scoop the mixture into mounds on a baking sheet, leaving space for each cookie to spread. Use a fork to flatten the top of each cookie. Bake for 10 minutes. Allow to cool on the tray for 5 minutes before transferring to a wire rack.

DARK CHOCOLATE AVOCADO MOUSSE

Serves 2

INGREDIENTS

2 tablespoons dark chocolate chips, melted

1 ripe avocado

3 tablespoons cocoa powder

2 tablespoons nondairy milk

¼ teaspoon pure vanilla extract

3 tablespoons erythritol, maple syrup, or sugar

Pinch salt

Place the chocolate chips (or several squares of dark chocolate) in a small microwave-safe bowl and microwave in 10-second increments until just melted. Transfer the melted chocolate to a food processor or blender along with the remaining ingredients and process until smooth. Serve immediately or enjoy frozen.

CHERRY BANANA ICE CREAM

Serves 2

INGREDIENTS

2 frozen bananas

1 cup frozen cherries or strawberries

2 tablespoons avocado oil

¼ cup water or nondairy milk

Pinch salt

Peel the bananas, cut them into 1-inch slices, and freeze for at least several hours or overnight. Transfer the frozen bananas to a high-powered blender or food processor along with the remaining ingredients. Blend until smooth, scraping down the sides as needed. Serve immediately.

BLUEBERRY ALMOND CAKE

Serves 8

INGREDIENTS

4 large eggs

¼ cup avocado or safflower oil

2 tablespoons water or milk of choice

1 tablespoon pure vanilla extract

1 teaspoon pure almond extract

½ cup sugar or erythritol

1½ cups blanched almond flour, plus 1 tablespoon

1 teaspoon baking powder

½ teaspoon baking soda

½ teaspoon ground cinnamon

½ teaspoon salt

1 cup fresh or frozen blueberries

Preheat the oven to 325°F (165°C). Grease an 8-inch square baking pan.

Using an electric mixer or whisk, beat the eggs with the oil, water, vanilla, almond extract, and sugar. In a separate bowl, combine 1½ cups of almond flour with the baking powder, baking soda, cinnamon, and salt. Pour the wet ingredients into the dry ingredients and stir to combine. Toss half the blueberries with the remaining 1 tablespoon of almond flour (to prevent the berries sinking). Gently fold the blueberries into the batter. Transfer the batter to the baking pan. Top with the remaining blueberries, gently them pressing into the batter. Bake until the center is firm to the touch, and a toothpick inserted in the center comes out clean, about 35 minutes.

CHICKPEA COOKIE DOUGH

INGREDIENTS

1 cup cooked chickpeas*

3 tablespoons cashew, peanut, or sunflower seed butter

1 teaspoon pure vanilla extract

¼ teaspoon salt

⅛ teaspoon baking soda

3 tablespoons almond flour or ground flaxseed

1 to **2** tablespoons erythritol or maple syrup

1 to **2** tablespoons water or milk of choice, if needed

¼ cup chocolate chips

Combine the chickpeas, nut butter, vanilla, salt, baking soda, flour, and sweetener in a food processor. Process until very smooth, scraping the sides and adding water if needed. Transfer to a bowl and mix in the chocolate chips.

*This recipe works much better with chickpeas that have been soaked overnight and pressure cooked for 20 minutes. If using canned chickpeas, rinse them very well and boil for 5 to 10 minutes to ensure a creamy consistency.

LEMON AND ALMOND COOKIES

INGREDIENTS

2 large eggs

½ cup honey

⅓ cup erythritol

1 teaspoon pure vanilla extract

1 to **2** teaspoons lemon zest

3½ cups blanched almond flour

1 cup slivered almonds

Preheat the oven to 300°F (150°C). Using an electric mixer, beat together the eggs, honey, erythritol, vanilla, and lemon zest. Add the almond flour and beat until combined into a smooth paste. Form the dough into 1-inch-diameter balls. Roughly chop the slivered almonds and spread them out on a plate or cutting board. Roll the dough balls in the almonds then transfer to a baking sheet . Bake for 12 to 15 minutes.

GINGERBREAD MUG CAKE

Serves 1

INGREDIENTS

1 egg

1 tablespoon water

1 tablespoon avocado or safflower oil

teaspoon pure vanilla extract

¼ teaspoon ground ginger

¼ teaspoon ground cinnamon

2 tablespoons almond flour or gluten-free flour

1 tablespoon coconut flour

½ teaspoon baking powder

2 teaspoons sugar or erythritol

In a small mixing bowl, whisk together the egg, water, oil, vanilla, ginger, and cinnamon. Add the remaining ingredients and mix with a fork until the batter is smooth. Pour the batter into a microwave-safe mug and microwave for 1 minute. If the top of the cake is not yet firm, microwave for an additional 15 to 30 seconds.

BERRY COMPOTE

Serves 2 to 4

INGREDIENTS

1 ripe pear, grated or finely chopped

½ teaspoon pure vanilla extract

1 cup frozen blueberries, divided

1 cup frozen blackberries, divided

1 tablespoon freshly squeezed lemon juice

Combine the pear, vanilla, half the blueberries, and half the blackberries in a microwave-safe bowl. Microwave for 5 minutes. Stir in the remaining berries and lemon juice and microwave for an additional 1 minute. The compote will thicken slightly as it cools. For an even thicker consistency, add 1 tablespoon of gelatin mixed with ¼ cup of water to the berries before microwaving.

POMEGRANATE JELLY

Serves 8

INGREDIENTS

2 tablespoons gelatin

1½ cups pomegranate juice, divided

1 cup boiling water

Bloom the gelatin in ½ cup of pomegranate juice. Add the boiling water and stir to combine. When the gelatin is fully dissolved, stir in the remaining 1 cup of pomegranate juice. Pour into a rectangular baking dish or individual serving bowls. Refrigerate until set (1 to 2 hours).

MELON MINT SALAD

Serves 2 to 4

INGREDIENTS

1 to **2** tablespoons freshly squeezed lime juice

1 tablespoon olive oil

2 cups cubed honeydew melon

2 tablespoons chopped fresh mint leaves

1 teaspoon grated lime zest

Pour the lime juice and olive oil over the melon, add the mint and lime zest, and toss to combine.

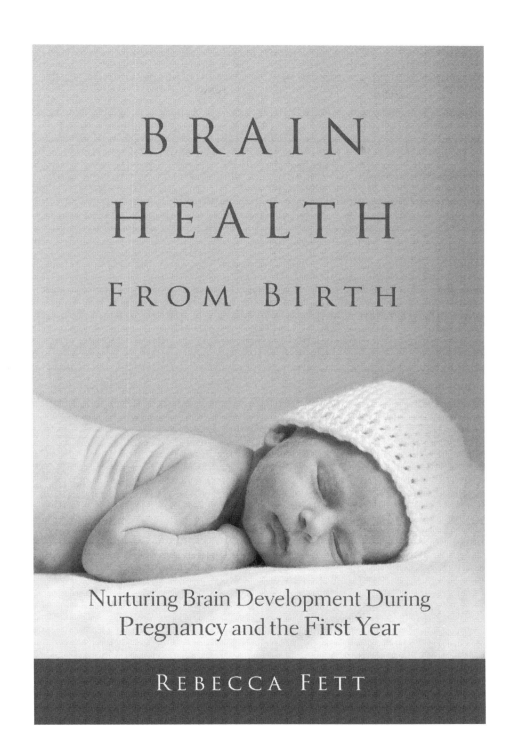

BRAIN HEALTH

FROM BIRTH

Nurturing Brain Development During
Pregnancy and the First Year

REBECCA FETT

References

1   Gaskins, A. J., Nassan, F. L., Chiu, Y. H., Arvizu, M., Williams, P. L., Keller, M.
    G.,...& EARTH Study Team. (2019). Dietary patterns and outcomes of assisted
    reproduction. American journal of obstetrics and gynecology, 220(6), 567-e1.
    Karayiannis, D., Kontogianni, M. D., Mendorou, C., Mastrominas, M., & Yianna-
    kouris, N. (2018). Adherence to the Mediterranean diet and IVF success rate among
    non-obese women attempting fertility. Human Reproduction, 33(3), 494-502.

2   Karayiannis, D., Kontogianni, M. D., Mendorou, C., Mastrominas, M., & Yianna-
    kouris, N. (2018). Adherence to the Mediterranean diet and IVF success rate among
    non-obese women attempting fertility. Human Reproduction, 33(3), 494-502.

3   Koloverou, E., Panagiotakos, D. B., Pitsavos, C., Chrysohoou, C., Georgousopoulou,
    E. N., Grekas, A.,...& Stefanadis, C. (2016). Adherence to Mediterranean diet and
    10–year incidence (2002–2012) of diabetes: correlations with inflammatory and
    oxidative stress biomarkers in the ATTICA cohort study. Diabetes/metabolism
    research and reviews, 32(1), 73-81.

4   Karayiannis, D., Kontogianni, M. D., Mendorou, C., Mastrominas, M., & Yianna-
    kouris, N. (2018). Adherence to the Mediterranean diet and IVF success rate among
    non-obese women attempting fertility. Human Reproduction, 33(3), 494-502.

5   Nicolau, P., Miralpeix, E., Sola, I., Carreras, R., & Checa, M. A. (2014). Alcohol con-
    sumption and in vitro fertilization: a review of the literature. Gynecological Endo-
    crinology, 30(11), 759-763.

6   Lyngsø, J., Ramlau-Hansen, C. H., Bay, B., Ingerslev, H. J., Strandberg-Larsen, K., &
    Kesmodel, U. S. (2019). Low-to-moderate alcohol consumption and success in fer-
    tility treatment: a Danish cohort study. Human Reproduction, 34(7), 1334-1344.

7   Avalos, L. A., Roberts, S. C., Kaskutas, L. A., Block, G., & Li, D. K. (2014). Volume
    and type of alcohol during early pregnancy and the risk of miscarriage. Substance
    use & misuse, 49(11), 1437-1445.
    Sundermann, A. C., Zhao, S., Young, C. L., Lam, L., Jones, S. H., Velez Edwards,
    D. R., & Hartmann, K. E. (2019). Alcohol Use in Pregnancy and Miscarriage: A
    Systematic Review and Meta-Analysis. Alcoholism: Clinical and Experimental
    Research, 43(8), 1606-1616.

8   Machtinger, R., Gaskins, A. J., Mansur, A., Adir, M., Racowsky, C., Baccarelli, A.
    A.,...& Chavarro, J. E. (2017). Association between preconception maternal beverage
    intake and in vitro fertilization outcomes. Fertility and sterility, 108(6), 1026-1033.

9   Ghosh, I., Sharma, P. K., Rahman, M., & Lahkar, K. (2019). Sugar-sweetened bev-
    erage intake in relation to semen quality in infertile couples– a prospective observa-
    tional study. Fertility Science and Research, 6(1), 40.

10 Russell, J. B., Abboud, C., Williams, A., Gibbs, M., Pritchard, S., & Chal-
    fant, D. (2012). Does changing a patient's dietary consumption of proteins and

carbohydrates impact blastocyst development and clinical pregnancy rates from one cycle to the next?. Fertility and Sterility, 98(3), S47.

11   Chiu, Y. H., Afeiche, M. C., Gaskins, A. J., Williams, P. L., Petrozza, J. C., Tanrikut, C.,...& Chavarro, J. E. (2015). Fruit and vegetable intake and their pesticide residues in relation to semen quality among men from a fertility clinic. *Human Reproduction*, 30(6), 1342-1351.

12   Bouzari, A., Holstege, D., & Barrett, D. M. (2015). Vitamin retention in eight fruits and vegetables: a comparison of refrigerated and frozen storage. *Journal of agricultural and food chemistry*, 63(3), 957-962.

13   http://www.noarthritis.com/nightshades.htm

14   Afifi, L., Danesh, M. J., Lee, K. M., Beroukhim, K., Farahnik, B., Ahn, R. S.,...& Liao, W. (2017). Dietary behaviors in psoriasis: patient-reported outcomes from a US National Survey. *Dermatology and therapy*, 7(2), 227-242.

15   Patel, B., Schutte, R., Sporns, P., Doyle, J., Jewel, L., & Fedorak, R. N. (2002). Potato glycoalkaloids adversely affect intestinal permeability and aggravate inflammatory bowel disease. Inflammatory bowel diseases, 8(5), 340-346.
      Hashimoto, K., Kawagishi, H., Nakayama, T., & Shimizu, M. (1997). Effect of capsianoside, a diterpene glycoside, on tight-junctional permeability. Biochimica et Biophysica Acta (BBA)-Biomembranes, 1323(2), 281-290.
      Pramod, S. N., Venkatesh, Y. P., & Mahesh, P. A. (2007). Potato lectin activates basophils and mast cells of atopic subjects by its interaction with core chitobiose of cell-bound non-specific immunoglobulin E. Clinical & Experimental Immunology, 148(3), 391-401.

16   Shukla, A. P., Iliescu, R. G., Thomas, C. E., & Aronne, L. J. (2015). Food order has a significant impact on postprandial glucose and insulin levels. Diabetes care, 38(7), e98-e99

17   Koloverou, E., Panagiotakos, D. B., Pitsavos, C., Chrysohoou, C., Georgousopoulou, E. N., Grekas, A.,...& Stefanadis, C. (2016). Adherence to Mediterranean diet and 10–year incidence (2002–2012) of diabetes: correlations with inflammatory and oxidative stress biomarkers in the ATTICA cohort study. Diabetes/metabolism research and reviews, 32(1), 73-81.

18   Willis, S. K., Wise, L. A., Wesselink, A. K., Rothman, K., Tucker, K. L., & Hatch, E. E. (2018). Glycemic load, dietary fiber, and added sugar and fecundability in a North American preconception cohort. Fertility and Sterility, 110(4), e95.
      Willis, S. K., Wise, L. A., Wesselink, A. K., Rothman, K. J., Mikkelsen, E. M., Tucker, K. L.,...& Hatch, E. E. (2020). Glycemic load, dietary fiber, and added sugar and fecundability in 2 preconception cohorts. The American Journal of Clinical Nutrition.

19   Chavarro, J. E., Rich-Edwards, J. W., Rosner, B. A., & Willett, W. C. (2009). A prospective study of dietary carbohydrate quantity and quality in relation to risk of ovulatory infertility. European journal of clinical nutrition, 63(1), 78-86.

20   Grieger, J. A., Grzeskowiak, L. E., Bianco-Miotto, T., Jankovic-Karasoulos, T., Moran, L. J., Wilson, R. L.,...& Myers, J. (2018). Pre-pregnancy fast food and fruit intake is associated with time to pregnancy. Human Reproduction, 33(6), 1063-1070.

21   Fedder, M. D., Jakobsen, H. B., Giversen, I., Christensen, L. P., Parner, E. T., & Fedder, J. (2014). An extract of pomegranate fruit and galangal rhizome increases the numbers of motile sperm: a prospective, randomised, controlled, double-blinded trial. PloS one, 9(10).

22   De Punder, K., & Pruimboom, L. (2013). The dietary intake of wheat and other cereal grains and their role in inflammation. Nutrients, 5(3), 771-787.
Shibasaki, M., Sumazaki, R., Isoyama, S., & Takita, H. (1992). Interaction of lectins with human IgE: IgE-binding property and histamine-releasing activity of twelve plant lectins. International archives of allergy and immunology, 98(1), 18-25.
Nachbar, M. S., & Oppenheim, J. D. (1980). Lectins in the United States diet: a survey of lectins in commonly consumed foods and a review of the literature. The American journal of clinical nutrition, 33(11), 2338-2345;
Matucci, A., Veneri, G., Dalla Pellegrina, C., Zoccatelli, G., Vincenzi, S., Chignola, R., ... & Rizzi, C. (2004). Temperature-dependent decay of wheat germ agglutinin activity and its implications for food processing and analysis. Food Control, 15(5), 391-395.
Rizzi, C., Galeoto, L., Zoccatelli, G., Vincenzi, S., Chignola, R., & Peruffo, A. D. (2003). Active soybean lectin in foods: quantitative determination by ELISA using immobilised asialofetuin. Food research international, 36(8), 815-821.
Pramod, S. N., Venkatesh, Y. P., & Mahesh, P. A. (2007). Potato lectin activates basophils and mast cells of atopic subjects by its interaction with core chitobiose of cell-bound non-specific immunoglobulin E. Clinical & Experimental Immunology, 148(3), 391-401

23   Pan, L., Qin, G., Zhao, Y., Wang, J., Liu, F., & Che, D. (2013). Effects of soybean agglutinin on mechanical barrier function and tight junction protein expression in intestinal epithelial cells from piglets. International journal of molecular sciences, 14(11), 21689-21704.
Nachbar, M. S., & Oppenheim, J. D. (1980). Lectins in the United States diet: a survey of lectins in commonly consumed foods and a review of the literature. The American journal of clinical nutrition, 33(11), 2338-2345;
Pusztai, A., & Bardocz, S. (1996). Biological effects of plant lectins on the gastro-intestinal tract: metabolic consequences and applications. Trends in glycoscience and glycotechnology, 8, 149-166.
Dalla Pellegrina, C., Perbellini, O., Scupoli, M. T., Tomelleri, C., Zanetti, C., Zoccatelli, G., ... & Chignola, R. (2009). Effects of wheat germ agglutinin on human gastrointestinal epithelium: insights from an experimental model of immune/epithelial cell interaction. Toxicology and applied pharmacology, 237(2), 146-153
Pan, L., Qin, G., Zhao, Y., Wang, J., Liu, F., & Che, D. (2013). Effects of soybean agglutinin on mechanical barrier function and tight junction protein expression in intestinal epithelial cells from piglets. International journal of molecular sciences, 14(11), 21689-21704.

24   Messina, V. (2014). Nutritional and health benefits of dried beans. The American journal of clinical nutrition, 100(Supplement 1), 437S-442S.

25   Carlini, C. R., & Udedibie, A. B. (1997). Comparative effects of processing methods on hemagglutinating and antitryptic activities of Canavalia ensiformis and Canavalia braziliensis seeds. Journal of Agricultural and Food Chemistry, 45(11), 4372-4377.

26   Thomson, L. U., Rea, R. L., & Jenkins, D. J. (1983). Effect of heat processing on hemagglutinin activity in red kidney beans. Journal of Food Science, 48(1), 235-236. Carlini, C. R., & Udedibie, A. B. (1997). Comparative effects of processing methods on hemagglutinating and antitryptic activities of Canavalia ensiformis and Canavalia braziliensis seeds. Journal of Agricultural and Food Chemistry, 45(11), 4372-4377.

27   Barrea, L., Balato, N., Di Somma, C., Macchia, P. E., Napolitano, M., Savanelli, M. C.,…& Savastano, S. (2015). Nutrition and psoriasis: is there any association between the severity of the disease and adherence to the Mediterranean diet?. Journal of translational medicine, 13(1), 18. Saraf-Bank, S., Esmaillzadeh, A., Faghihimani, E., & Azadbakht, L. (2015). Effect of non-soy legume consumption on inflammation and serum adiponectin levels among first-degree relatives of patients with diabetes: A randomized, crossover study. Nutrition, 31(3), 459-465.

28   Alwahab, U. A., Pantalone, K. M., & Burguera, B. (2018). A ketogenic diet may restore fertility in women with polycystic ovary syndrome: A case series. AACE Clinical Case Reports, 4(5), e427-e431.

29   Paoli, A., Mancin, L., Giacona, M. C., Bianco, A., & Caprio, M. (2020). Effects of a ketogenic diet in overweight women with polycystic ovary syndrome. Journal of Translational Medicine, 18(1), 1-11. Mavropoulos, J. C., Yancy, W. S., Hepburn, J., & Westman, E. C. (2005). The effects of a low-carbohydrate, ketogenic diet on the polycystic ovary syndrome: a pilot study. Nutrition & metabolism, 2(1), 35. Douglas, C. C., Gower, B. A., Darnell, B. E., Ovalle, F., Oster, R. A., & Azziz, R. (2006). Role of diet in the treatment of polycystic ovary syndrome. Fertility and sterility, 85(3), 679-688.

30   Stimson, R. H., Johnstone, A. M., Homer, N. Z., Wake, D. J., Morton, N. M., Andrew, R.,…& Walker, B. R. (2007). Dietary macronutrient content alters cortisol metabolism independently of body weight changes in obese men. The Journal of Clinical Endocrinology & Metabolism, 92(11), 4480-4484. Grandl, G., Straub, L., Rudigier, C., Arnold, M., Wueest, S., Konrad, D., & Wolfrum, C. (2018). Short-term feeding of a ketogenic diet induces more severe hepatic insulin resistance than an obesogenic high-fat diet. The Journal of physiology, 596(19), 4597-4609. Jornayvaz, F. R., Jurczak, M. J., Lee, H. Y., Birkenfeld, A. L., Frederick, D. W., Zhang, D.,…& Shulman, G. I. (2010). A high-fat, ketogenic diet causes hepatic insulin resistance in mice, despite increasing energy expenditure and preventing weight gain. American Journal of Physiology-Endocrinology and Metabolism, 299(5), E808-E815.

31   McGrice, M., & Porter, J. (2017). The effect of low carbohydrate diets on fertility hormones and outcomes in overweight and obese women: a systematic review. Nutrients, 9(3), 204.

32   Mehrabani, H. H., Salehpour, S., Amiri, Z., Farahani, S. J., Meyer, B. J., & Tahbaz, F. (2012). Beneficial effects of a high-protein, low-glycemic-load hypocaloric diet in overweight and obese women with polycystic ovary syndrome: a randomized controlled intervention study. Journal of the American College of Nutrition, 31(2), 117-125.
Moran, L. J., Ko, H., Misso, M., Marsh, K., Noakes, M., Talbot, M.,... & Teede, H. J. (2013). Dietary composition in the treatment of polycystic ovary syndrome: a systematic review to inform evidence-based guidelines. Journal of the Academy of Nutrition and Dietetics, 113(4), 520-545.

33   Mady, M. A., Kossoff, E. H., McGregor, A. L., Wheless, J. W., Pyzik, P. L., & Freeman, J. M. (2003). The ketogenic diet: adolescents can do it, too. Epilepsia, 44(6), 847-851.

34   Mathieson, R. A., Walberg, J. L., Gwazdauskas, F. C., Hinkle, D. E., & Gregg, J. M. (1986). The effect of varying carbohydrate content of a very-low-caloric diet on resting metabolic rate and thyroid hormones. Metabolism, 35(5), 394-398.
Kose, E., Guzel, O., Demir, K., & Arslan, N. (2017). Changes of thyroid hormonal status in patients receiving ketogenic diet due to intractable epilepsy. Journal of Pediatric Endocrinology and Metabolism, 30(4), 411-416.

35   Harvie, M. N., Pegington, M., Mattson, M. P., Frystyk, J., Dillon, B., Evans, G.,... & Son, T. G. (2011). The effects of intermittent or continuous energy restriction on weight loss and metabolic disease risk markers: a randomized trial in young overweight women. International journal of obesity, 35(5), 714-727.
Bergendahl, M., Evans, W. S., Pastor, C., Patel, A., Iranmanesh, A., & Veldhuis, J. D. (1999). Short-term fasting suppresses leptin and (conversely) activates disorderly growth hormone secretion in midluteal phase women—a clinical research center study. The Journal of Clinical Endocrinology & Metabolism, 84(3), 883-894.
Perakakis, N., Upadhyay, J., Ghaly, W., Chen, J., Chrysafi, P., Anastasilakis, A. D., & Mantzoros, C. S. (2018). Regulation of the activins-follistatins-inhibins axis by energy status: Impact on reproductive function. Metabolism, 85, 240-249.

36   Pieczyńska, J. (2018). Do celiac disease and non-celiac gluten sensitivity have the same effects on reproductive disorders?. Nutrition, 48, 18-23.

37   Ahmed, S. H., Guillem, K., & Vandaele, Y. (2013). Sugar addiction: pushing the drug-sugar analogy to the limit. Current Opinion in Clinical Nutrition & Metabolic Care, 16(4), 434-439.

38   Al-Saleh, A. M., Corkey, B., Deeney, J., Tornheim, K., & Bauer, E. (2011). Effect of artificial sweeteners on insulin secretion, ROS, and oxygen consumption in pancreatic beta cells.

39   Setti, A. S., Braga, D. P. D. A. F., Halpern, G., Rita de Cássia, S. F., Iaconelli Jr, A., & Borges Jr, E. (2018). Is there an association between artificial sweetener consumption and assisted reproduction outcomes?. Reproductive biomedicine online, 36(2), 145-153.

40   Rahimipour, M., Talebi, A. R., Anvari, M., Sarcheshmeh, A. A., & Omidi, M. (2014). Saccharin consumption increases sperm DNA fragmentation and apoptosis in mice. Iranian journal of reproductive medicine, 12(5), 307.

41   Melis, M. S. (1999). Effects of chronic administration of Stevia rebaudiana on fertility in rats. Journal of ethnopharmacology, 67(2), 157-161.
Shannon, M., Rehfeld, A., Frizzell, C., Livingstone, C., McGonagle, C., Skakkebaek, N. E.,...& Connolly, L. (2016). In vitro bioassay investigations of the endocrine disrupting potential of steviol glycosides and their metabolite steviol, components of the natural sweetener Stevia. Molecular and cellular endocrinology, 427, 65-72.

42   Allgrove, J., Farrell, E., Gleeson, M., Williamson, G., & Cooper, K. (2011). Regular dark chocolate consumption's reduction of oxidative stress and increase of free-fatty-acid mobilization in response to prolonged cycling. International journal of sport nutrition and exercise metabolism, 21(2), 113-123.
Nanetti, L., Raffaelli, F., Tranquilli, A. L., Fiorini, R., Mazzanti, L., & Vignini, A. (2012). Effect of consumption of dark chocolate on oxidative stress in lipoproteins and platelets in women and in men. Appetite, 58(1), 400-405.
Engler, M. B., & Engler, M. M. (2006). The emerging role of flavonoid-rich cocoa and chocolate in cardiovascular health and disease. Nutrition reviews, 64(3), 109-118.

43   Wise, P. M., Nattress, L., Flammer, L. J., & Beauchamp, G. K. (2016). Reduced dietary intake of simple sugars alters perceived sweet taste intensity but not perceived pleasantness. The American journal of clinical nutrition, 103(1), 50-60.

44   Bartolotto, C. (2015). Does consuming sugar and artificial sweeteners change taste preferences?. The Permanente Journal, 19(3), 81.

45   Alcock, J., Maley, C. C., & Aktipis, C. A. (2014). Is eating behavior manipulated by the gastrointestinal microbiota? Evolutionary pressures and potential mechanisms. Bioessays, 36(10), 940-949.

46   Allonsius, C. N., van den Broek, M. F., De Boeck, I., Kiekens, S., Oerlemans, E. F., Kiekens, F.,...& Lebeer, S. (2017). Interplay between Lactobacillus rhamnosus GG and Candida and the involvement of exopolysaccharides. Microbial biotechnology, 10(6), 1753-1763.

47   Helmrich, S. P., Ragland, D. R., Leung, R. W., & Paffenbarger Jr, R. S. (1991). Physical activity and reduced occurrence of non-insulin-dependent diabetes mellitus. New England journal of medicine, 325(3), 147-152.

48   Lee, J. (2020). Determining the association between physical activity prior to conception and pregnancy rate: A systematic review and meta-analysis of prospective cohort studies. Health Care for Women International, 41(1), 38-53.
Wise, L. A., Rothman, K. J., Mikkelsen, E. M., Sørensen, H. T., Riis, A. H., & Hatch, E. E. (2012). A prospective cohort study of physical activity and time to pregnancy. Fertility and sterility, 97(5), 1136-1142.

49   Palomba, S., Falbo, A., Valli, B., Morini, D., Villani, M. T., Nicoli, A., & La Sala, G. B. (2014). Physical activity before IVF and ICSI cycles in infertile obese women: an observational cohort study. Reproductive biomedicine online, 29(1), 72-79.
Rao, M., Zeng, Z., & Tang, L. (2018). Maternal physical activity before IVF/ICSI cycles improves clinical pregnancy rate and live birth rate: a systematic review and meta-analysis. Reproductive Biology and Endocrinology, 16(1), 11.

Harrison, C. L., Lombard, C. B., Moran, L. J., & Teede, H. J. (2011). Exercise therapy in polycystic ovary syndrome: a systematic review. Human reproduction update, 17(2), 171-183.

50   Rao, M., Zeng, Z., & Tang, L. (2018). Maternal physical activity before IVF/ICSI cycles improves clinical pregnancy rate and live birth rate: a systematic review and meta-analysis. Reproductive Biology and Endocrinology, 16(1), 11.

Evenson, K. R., Calhoun, K. C., Herring, A. H., Pritchard, D., Wen, F., & Steiner, A. Z. (2014). Association of physical activity in the past year and immediately after in vitro fertilization on pregnancy. Fertility and sterility, 101(4), 1047-1054.

51   Gudmundsdottir, S. L., Flanders, W. D., & Augestad, L. B. (2009). Physical activity and fertility in women: the North-Trøndelag Health Study. Human Reproduction, 24(12), 3196-3204.

Wise, L. A., Rothman, K. J., Mikkelsen, E. M., Sørensen, H. T., Riis, A. H., & Hatch, E. E. (2012). A prospective cohort study of physical activity and time to pregnancy. Fertility and sterility, 97(5), 1136-1142.

52   Craciunas, L., & Tsampras, N. (2016). Bed rest following embryo transfer might negatively affect the outcome of IVF/ICSI: a systematic review and meta-analysis. Human Fertility, 19(1), 16-22.

Orvieto, R., Ashkenazi, J., Bar-Hava, I., & Ben-Rafael, Z. (1998). Bed rest following embryo transfer—necessary. Fertil Steril, 70(5), 982.

Botta, G., & Grudzinskas, G. (1997). Is a prolonged bed rest following embryo transfer useful?. Human Reproduction, 12(11), 2489-2492.

53   Wise, L. A., Cramer, D. W., Hornstein, M. D., Ashby, R. K., & Missmer, S. A. (2011). Physical activity and semen quality among men attending an infertility clinic. Fertility and sterility, 95(3), 1025-1030.

Kipandula, W., & Lampiao, F. (2015). Semen profiles of young men involved as bicycle taxi cyclists in Mangochi District, Malawi: A case-control study. Malawi Medical Journal, 27(4), 151-153.

Palekar, S. S., Karanje, N. V., & Palekar, S. S. (2016). A study on semen profile in bicycle cyclists. Indian Journal of Clinical Anatomy and Physiology, 3(4), 490-493.

54   Leibovitch, I., & Mor, Y. (2005). The vicious cycling: bicycling related urogenital disorders. European urology, 47(3), 277-287.

55   Arciero, P. J., Gentile, C. L., Pressman, R., Everett, M., Ormsbee, M. J., Martin, J.,…& Nindl, B. C. (2008). Moderate protein intake improves total and regional body composition and insulin sensitivity in overweight adults. Metabolism, 57(6), 757-765.

56   Chavarro, J. E., Rich-Edwards, J. W., Rosner, B. A., & Willett, W. C. (2008). Protein intake and ovulatory infertility. American journal of obstetrics and gynecology, 198(2), 210-e1.

57   Braga, D. P. A. F., Halpern, G., Setti, A. S., Figueira, R. C. S., Iaconelli Jr, A., & Borges Jr, E. (2015). The impact of food intake and social habits on embryo quality and the likelihood of blastocyst formation. Reproductive biomedicine online, 31(1), 30-38.

58   Eslamian, G., Amirjannati, N., Rashidkhani, B., Sadeghi, M. R., & Hekmatdoost, A. (2012). Intake of food groups and idiopathic asthenozoospermia: a case–control study. Human reproduction, 27(11), 3328-3336.
Gaskins, A. J., Colaci, D. S., Mendiola, J., Swan, S. H., & Chavarro, J. E. (2012). Dietary patterns and semen quality in young men. Human reproduction, 27(10), 2899-2907.
Afeiche, M. C., Gaskins, A. J., Williams, P. L., Toth, T. L., Wright, D. L., Tanrikut, C., ... & Chavarro, J. E. (2014). Processed meat intake is unfavorably and fish intake favorably associated with semen quality indicators among men attending a fertility clinic. The Journal of nutrition, 144(7), 1091-1098.
Mendiola, J., Torres-Cantero, A. M., Moreno-Grau, J. M., Ten, J., Roca, M., Moreno-Grau, S., & Bernabeu, R. (2009). Food intake and its relationship with semen quality: a case-control study. Fertility and sterility, 91(3), 812-818.

59   Jensen, T. K., Heitmann, B. L., Jensen, M. B., Halldorsson, T. I., Andersson, A. M., Skakkebæk, N. E., ... & Lassen, T. H. (2013). High dietary intake of saturated fat is associated with reduced semen quality among 701 young Danish men from the general population. The American journal of clinical nutrition, 97(2), 411-418.

60   Xia, W., Chiu, Y. H., Williams, P. L., Gaskins, A. J., Toth, T. L., Tanrikut, C., ... & Chavarro, J. E. (2015). Men's meat intake and treatment outcomes among couples undergoing assisted reproduction. Fertility and sterility, 104(4), 972-979.

61   Braga, D. P. A. F., Halpern, G., Setti, A. S., Figueira, R. C. S., Iaconelli Jr, A., & Borges Jr, E. (2015). The impact of food intake and social habits on embryo quality and the likelihood of blastocyst formation. Reproductive biomedicine online, 31(1), 30-38.
Nassan, F. L., Chiu, Y. H., Vanegas, J. C., Gaskins, A. J., Williams, P. L., Ford, J. B., ... & EARTH Study Team. (2018). Intake of protein-rich foods in relation to outcomes of infertility treatment with assisted reproductive technologies. The American journal of clinical nutrition, 108(5), 1104-1112.

62   Afeiche, M. C., Bridges, N. D., Williams, P. L., Gaskins, A. J., Tanrikut, C., Petrozza, J. C., ... & Chavarro, J. E. (2014). Dairy intake and semen quality among men attending a fertility clinic. Fertility and sterility, 101(5), 1280-1287.
Afeiche, M. C., Gaskins, A. J., Williams, P. L., Toth, T. L., Wright, D. L., Tanrikut, C., ... & Chavarro, J. E. (2014). Processed meat intake is unfavorably and fish intake favorably associated with semen quality indicators among men attending a fertility clinic. The Journal of nutrition, 144(7), 1091-1098.
Eslamian, G., Amirjannati, N., Rashidkhani, B., Sadeghi, M. R., & Hekmatdoost, A. (2012). Intake of food groups and idiopathic asthenozoospermia: a case–control study. Human reproduction, 27(11), 3328-3336.

63   Gaskins, A. J., Sundaram, R., Louis, B., Germaine, M., & Chavarro, J. E. (2018). Seafood intake, sexual activity, and time to pregnancy. The Journal of Clinical Endocrinology & Metabolism, 103(7), 2680-2688.

64   Vujkovic, M., de Vries, J. H., Lindemans, J., Macklon, N. S., van der Spek, P. J., Steegers, E. A., & Steegers-Theunissen, R. P. (2010). The preconception Mediterranean dietary pattern in couples undergoing in vitro fertilization/intracytoplasmic sperm injection treatment increases the chance of pregnancy. Fertility and sterility, 94(6), 2096-2101.

65   Wise, L. A., Wesselink, A. K., Tucker, K. L., Saklani, S., Mikkelsen, E. M., Cueto, H.,...& Rothman, K. J. (2018). Dietary fat intake and fecundability in 2 preconception cohort studies. American journal of epidemiology, 187(1), 60-74.

66   Chiu, Y. H., Karmon, A. E., Gaskins, A. J., Arvizu, M., Williams, P. L., Souter, I.,...& EARTH Study Team. (2018). Serum omega-3 fatty acids and treatment outcomes among women undergoing assisted reproduction. Human Reproduction, 33(1), 156-165.

67   Mirabi, P., Chaichi, M. J., Esmaeilzadeh, S., Jorsaraei, S. G. A., Bijani, A., Ehsani, M., & hashemi Karooee, S. F. (2017). The role of fatty acids on ICSI outcomes: a prospective cohort study. Lipids in health and disease, 16(1), 18.
      Kim, C. H., Yoon, J. W., Ahn, J. W., Kang, H. J., Lee, J. W., & Kang, B. M. (2010). The effect of supplementation with omega-3-polyunsaturated fatty acids in intracytoplasmic sperm injection cycles for infertile patients with a history of unexplained total fertilization failure. Fertility and Sterility, 94(4), S242.

68   González-Ravina, C., Aguirre-Lipperheide, M., Pinto, F., Martín-Lozano, D., Fernández-Sánchez, M., Blasco, V.,...& Candenas, L. (2018). Effect of dietary supplementation with a highly pure and concentrated docosahexaenoic acid (DHA) supplement on human sperm function. Reproductive biology, 18(3), 282-288.
      Martínez-Soto, J. C., Domingo, J. C., Cordobilla, B., Nicolás, M., Fernández, L., Albero, P.,...& Landeras, J. (2016). Dietary supplementation with docosahexaenoic acid (DHA) improves seminal antioxidant status and decreases sperm DNA fragmentation. Systems biology in reproductive medicine, 62(6), 387-395.
      Hosseini, B., Nourmohamadi, M., Hajipour, S., Taghizadeh, M., Asemi, Z., Keshavarz, S. A., & Jafarnejad, S. (2019). The effect of omega-3 fatty acids, EPA, and/or DHA on male infertility: a systematic review and meta-analysis. Journal of dietary supplements, 16(2), 245-256.

69   Nassan, F. L., Chiu, Y. H., Vanegas, J. C., Gaskins, A. J., Williams, P. L., Ford, J. B.,...& EARTH Study Team. (2018). Intake of protein-rich foods in relation to outcomes of infertility treatment with assisted reproductive technologies. The American journal of clinical nutrition, 108(5), 1104-1112.

70   Gerster, H. (1998). Can adults adequately convert a-linolenic acid (18: 3n-3) to eicosapentaenoic acid (20: 5n-3) and docosahexaenoic acid (22: 6n-3)?. International Journal for Vitamin and Nutrition Research, 68(3), 159-173.
      Lane, K., Derbyshire, E., Li, W., & Brennan, C. (2014). Bioavailability and potential uses of vegetarian sources of omega-3 fatty acids: a review of the literature. Critical reviews in food science and nutrition, 54(5), 572-579.

71   Blanchet, C., Lucas, M., Julien, P., Morin, R., Gingras, S., & Dewailly, É. (2005). Fatty acid composition of wild and farmed Atlantic salmon (Salmo salar) and rainbow trout (Oncorhynchus mykiss). Lipids, 40(5), 529-531.

72   da Costa, K. A., Gaffney, C. E., Fischer, L. M., & Zeisel, S. H. (2005). Choline deficiency in mice and humans is associated with increased plasma homocysteine concentration after a methionine load. The American journal of clinical nutrition, 81(2), 440-444.

73   Brunst, K. J., Wright, R. O., DiGioia, K., Enlow, M. B., Fernandez, H., Wright, R. J., & Kannan, S. (2014). Racial/ethnic and sociodemographic factors associated with

micronutrient intakes and inadequacies among pregnant women in an urban US population. *Public Health Nutrition, 17*(9), 1960–1970.

Wallace, T. C., & Fulgoni, V. L. (2017). Usual choline intakes are associated with egg and protein food consumption in the United States. *Nutrients, 9*(8), 839.

74   Jacobsen, B. K., Jaceldo-Siegl, K., Knutsen, S. F., Fan, J., Oda, K., & Fraser, G. E. (2014). Soy isoflavone intake and the likelihood of ever becoming a mother: the Adventist Health Study-2. International journal of women's health, 6, 377. This study is widely relied upon to argue negative impact of Soy. But it found found only a small difference in fertility among the women who consumed the most soy, with a 3% lower birth rate.

75   Vanegas, J. C., Afeiche, M. C., Gaskins, A. J., Mínguez-Alarcón, L., Williams, P. L., Wright, D. L.,… & Chavarro, J. E. (2015). Soy food intake and treatment outcomes of women undergoing assisted reproductive technology. Fertility and sterility, 103(3), 749-755.

76   Unfer, V., Casini, M. L., Gerli, S., Costabile, L., Mignosa, M., & Di Renzo, G. C. (2004). Phytoestrogens may improve the pregnancy rate in in vitro fertilization–embryo transfer cycles: a prospective, controlled, randomized trial. Fertility and sterility, 82(6), 1509-1513.

77   Chavarro, J. E., Rich-Edwards, J. W., Rosner, B. A., & Willett, W. C. (2008). Protein intake and ovulatory infertility. American journal of obstetrics and gynecology, 198(2), 210-e1.

78   Jamilian, M., & Asemi, Z. (2016). The effects of soy isoflavones on metabolic status of patients with polycystic ovary syndrome. The Journal of Clinical Endocrinology & Metabolism, 101(9), 3386-3394.

79   Chavarro, J. E., Toth, T. L., Sadio, S. M., & Hauser, R. (2008). Soy food and isoflavone intake in relation to semen quality parameters among men from an infertility clinic. Human reproduction, 23(11), 2584-2590.

80   Mínguez-Alarcón, L., Afeiche, M. C., Chiu, Y. H., Vanegas, J. C., Williams, P. L., Tanrikut, C.,… & Chavarro, J. E. (2015). Male soy food intake was not associated with in vitro fertilization outcomes among couples attending a fertility center. Andrology, 3(4), 702-708.

Beaton, L. K., McVeigh, B. L., Dillingham, B. L., Lampe, J. W., & Duncan, A. M. (2010). Soy protein isolates of varying isoflavone content do not adversely affect semen quality in healthy young men. Fertility and sterility, 94(5), 1717-1722.

81   Otun, J., Sahebkar, A., Östlundh, L., Atkin, S. L., & Sathyapalan, T. (2019). Systematic review and meta-analysis on the effect of soy on thyroid function. Scientific reports, 9(1), 1-9.

82   Otun, J., Sahebkar, A., Östlundh, L., Atkin, S. L., & Sathyapalan, T. (2019). Systematic review and meta-analysis on the effect of soy on thyroid function. Scientific reports, 9(1), 1-9.

83   Doerge, D. R., & Sheehan, D. M. (2002). Goitrogenic and estrogenic activity of soy isoflavones. Environmental health perspectives, 110(suppl 3), 349-353.

84   Vojdani, A. (2020). Reaction of food-specific antibodies with different tissue antigens. International Journal of Food Science & Technology, 55(4), 1800-1815.

85   Wise, L. A., Wesselink, A. K., Mikkelsen, E. M., Cueto, H., Hahn, K. A., Rothman, K. J.,... & Hatch, E. E. (2017). Dairy intake and fecundability in 2 preconception cohort studies. The American journal of clinical nutrition, 105(1), 100-110.
Chavarro, J. E., Rich-Edwards, J. W., Rosner, B., & Willett, W. C. (2007). A prospective study of dairy foods intake and anovulatory infertility. Human Reproduction, 22(5), 1340-1347.
Greenlee, A. R., Arbuckle, T. E., & Chyou, P. H. (2003). Risk factors for female infertility in an agricultural region. Epidemiology, 429-436.

86   Afeiche, M. C., Chiu, Y. H., Gaskins, A. J., Williams, P. L., Souter, I., Wright, D. L.,... & Chavarro, J. E. (2016). Dairy intake in relation to in vitro fertilization outcomes among women from a fertility clinic. Human Reproduction, 31(3), 563-571.

87   Wise, L. A., Wesselink, A. K., Mikkelsen, E. M., Cueto, H., Hahn, K. A., Rothman, K. J.,... & Hatch, E. E. (2017). Dairy intake and fecundability in 2 preconception cohort studies. The American journal of clinical nutrition, 105(1), 100-110.

88   Afeiche, M., Williams, P. L., Mendiola, J., Gaskins, A. J., Jørgensen, N., Swan, S. H., & Chavarro, J. E. (2013). Dairy food intake in relation to semen quality and reproductive hormone levels among physically active young men. Human reproduction, 28(8), 2265-2275.

89   Afeiche, M. C., Bridges, N. D., Williams, P. L., Gaskins, A. J., Tanrikut, C., Petrozza, J. C.,... & Chavarro, J. E. (2014). Dairy intake and semen quality among men attending a fertility clinic. Fertility and sterility, 101(5), 1280-1287.

90   Winger, E. E., Reed, J. L., Ashoush, S., El-Toukhy, T., & Taranissi, M. (2012). Die-Off Ratio Correlates with Increased TNF-α: IL-10 Ratio and Decreased IVF Success Rates Correctable with H umira. American Journal of Reproductive Immunology, 68(5), 428-437.

91   Maxia, N., Uccella, S., Ersettigh, G., Fantuzzi, M., Manganini, M., Scozzesi, A., & Colognato, R. (2018). Can unexplained infertility be evaluated by a new immunological four-biomarkers panel? A pilot study. Minerva ginecologica, 70(2), 129-137.
Xie, J., Yan, L., Cheng, Z., Qiang, L., Yan, J., Liu, Y.,... & Hao, C. (2018). Potential effect of inflammation on the failure risk of in vitro fertilization and embryo transfer among infertile women. Human Fertility, 1-9.
Buyuk, E., Asemota, O. A., Merhi, Z., Charron, M. J., Berger, D. S., Zapantis, A., & Jindal, S. K. (2017). Serum and follicular fluid monocyte chemotactic protein-1 levels are elevated in obese women and are associated with poorer clinical pregnancy rate after in vitro fertilization: a pilot study. Fertility and sterility, 107(3), 632-640.
Wagner, M. M., Jukema, J. W., Hermes, W., le Cessie, S., de Groot, C. J., Bakker, J. A.,... & Bloemenkamp, K. W. (2018). Assessment of novel cardiovascular biomarkers in women with a history of recurrent miscarriage. Pregnancy hypertension, 11, 129-135.
See also: Ahmed, S. K., Mahmood, N., Malalla, Z. H., Alsobyani, F. M., Al-Kiyumi, I. S., & Almawi, W. Y. (2015). C-reactive protein gene variants associated with recurrent pregnancy loss independent of CRP serum levels: a case-control study. Gene, 569(1), 136-140.

Kushnir, V. A., Solouki, S., Sarig-Meth, T., Vega, M. G., Albertini, D. F., Darmon, S. K.,...& Gleicher, N. (2016). Systemic inflammation and autoimmunity in women with chronic endometritis. American Journal of Reproductive Immunology, 75(6), 672-677.

92   Chrysohoou, C., Panagiotakos, D. B., Pitsavos, C., Das, U. N., & Stefanadis, C. (2004). Adherence to the Mediterranean diet attenuates inflammation and coagulation process in healthy adults: The ATTICA Study. Journal of the American College of Cardiology, 44(1), 152-158.

Richard, C., Couture, P., Desroches, S., & Lamarche, B. (2013). Effect of the Mediterranean diet with and without weight loss on markers of inflammation in men with metabolic syndrome. Obesity, 21(1), 51-57.

Sköldstam, L., Hagfors, L., & Johansson, G. (2003). An experimental study of a Mediterranean diet intervention for patients with rheumatoid arthritis. Annals of the rheumatic diseases, 62(3), 208-214.

93   Berbert, A. A., Kondo, C. R. M., Almendra, C. L., Matsuo, T., & Dichi, I. (2005). Supplementation of fish oil and olive oil in patients with rheumatoid arthritis. Nutrition, 21(2), 131-136.

Beauchamp, G. K., Keast, R. S., Morel, D., Lin, J., Pika, J., Han, Q.,...& Breslin, P. A. (2005). Phytochemistry: ibuprofen-like activity in extra-virgin olive oil. Nature, 437(7055), 45-46.

94   Bogani, P., Galli, C., Villa, M., & Visioli, F. (2007). Postprandial anti-inflammatory and antioxidant effects of extra virgin olive oil. Atherosclerosis, 190(1), 181-186.

95   Kremer, J. M., Lawrence, D. A., Jubiz, W., Digiacomo, R., Rynes, R., Bartholomew, L. E., & Sherman, M. (1990). Dietary fish oil and olive oil supplementation in patients with Rheumatoid Arthritis clinical and immunologic effects. Arthritis & Rheumatology, 33(6), 810-820.

96   Mumford, S. L., Browne, R. W., Kim, K., Nichols, C., Wilcox, B., Silver, R. M.,...& Perkins, N. J. (2018). Preconception plasma phospholipid fatty acids and fecundability. The Journal of Clinical Endocrinology & Metabolism, 103(12), 4501-4510.

97   Mirabi, P., Chaichi, M. J., Esmaeilzadeh, S., Jorsaraei, S. G. A., Bijani, A., Ehsani, M., & hashemi Karooee, S. F. (2017). The role of fatty acids on ICSI outcomes: a prospective cohort study. Lipids in health and disease, 16(1), 18.

98   Chavarro, J., Colaci, D., Afeiche, M., Gaskins, A., Wright, D., Toth, T., & Hauser, R. (2012). Dietary fat intake and in-vitro fertilization outcomes: saturated fat intake is associated with fewer metaphase 2 oocytes: O-200. Human Reproduction, 27.

99   Robbins, W. A., Xun, L., FitzGerald, L. Z., Esguerra, S., Henning, S. M., & Carpenter, C. L. (2012). Walnuts improve semen quality in men consuming a Western-style diet: randomized control dietary intervention trial. Biology of reproduction, 87(4), 101-1.

100 Salas-Huetos, A., Moraleda, R., Giardina, S., Anton, E., Blanco, J., Salas-Salvadó, J., & Bulló, M. (2018). Effect of nut consumption on semen quality and functionality in healthy men consuming a Western-style diet: a randomized controlled trial. The American journal of clinical nutrition, 108(5), 953-962.

101 Berbert, A. A., Kondo, C. R. M., Almendra, C. L., Matsuo, T., & Dichi, I. (2005). Supplementation of fish oil and olive oil in patients with rheumatoid arthritis. Nutrition, 21(2), 131-136.

102 Kermack, A. J., Lowen, P., Wellstead, S. J., Fisk, H. L., Montag, M., Cheong, Y., ... & Macklon, N. S. (2020). Effect of a 6-week "Mediterranean" dietary intervention on in vitro human embryo development: the Preconception Dietary Supplements in Assisted Reproduction double-blinded randomized controlled trial. Fertility and Sterility, 113(2), 260-269.

103 Dumas, J. A., Bunn, J. Y., Nickerson, J., Crain, K. I., Ebenstein, D. B., Tarleton, E. K., ... & Kien, C. L. (2016). Dietary saturated fat and monounsaturated fat have reversible effects on brain function and the secretion of pro-inflammatory cytokines in young women. Metabolism, 65(10), 1582-1588.
Kien, C. L., Bunn, J. Y., Fukagawa, N. K., Anathy, V., Matthews, D. E., Crain, K. I., ... & Poynter, M. E. (2015). Lipidomic evidence that lowering the typical dietary palmitate to oleate ratio in humans decreases the leukocyte production of proinflammatory cytokines and muscle expression of redox-sensitive genes. The Journal of nutritional biochemistry, 26(12), 1599-1606.
Ströher, D. J., de Oliveira, M. F., Martinez-Oliveira, P., Pilar, B. C., Cattelan, M. D. P., Rodrigues, E., ... & Manfredini, V. (2019). Virgin Coconut Oil Associated with High-Fat Diet Induces Metabolic Dysfunctions, Adipose Inflammation, and Hepatic Lipid Accumulation. Journal of Medicinal Food.

104 Lyte, J. M., Gabler, N. K., & Hollis, J. H. (2016). Postprandial serum endotoxin in healthy humans is modulated by dietary fat in a randomized, controlled, cross-over study. Lipids in Health and Disease, 15(1), 186.
Mani, V., Hollis, J. H., & Gabler, N. K. (2013). Dietary oil composition differentially modulates intestinal endotoxin transport and postprandial endotoxemia. Nutrition & metabolism, 10(1), 6.

105 Lyte, J. M., Gabler, N. K., & Hollis, J. H. (2016). Postprandial serum endotoxin in healthy humans is modulated by dietary fat in a randomized, controlled, cross-over study. Lipids in Health and Disease, 15(1), 186.
Mani, V., Hollis, J. H., & Gabler, N. K. (2013). Dietary oil composition differentially modulates intestinal endotoxin transport and postprandial endotoxemia. Nutrition & metabolism, 10(1), 6.

106 Mirabi, P., Chaichi, M. J., Esmaeilzadeh, S., Jorsaraei, S. G. A., Bijani, A., Ehsani, M., & hashemi Karooee, S. F. (2017). The role of fatty acids on ICSI outcomes: a prospective cohort study. Lipids in health and disease, 16(1), 18.
Chavarro, J., Colaci, D., Afeiche, M., Gaskins, A., Wright, D., Toth, T., & Hauser, R. (2012). Dietary fat intake and in-vitro fertilization outcomes: saturated fat intake is associated with fewer metaphase 2 oocytes: O-200. Human Reproduction, 27.

107 Mirabi, P., Chaichi, M. J., Esmaeilzadeh, S., Jorsaraei, S. G. A., Bijani, A., Ehsani, M., & hashemi Karooee, S. F. (2017). The role of fatty acids on ICSI outcomes: a prospective cohort study. Lipids in health and disease, 16(1), 18.

108 Ricci, E., Noli, S., Ferrari, S., La Vecchia, I., Castiglioni, M., Cipriani, S.,...& Agostoni, C. (2020). Fatty acids, food groups and semen variables in men referring to an Italian Fertility Clinic: Cross-sectional analysis of a prospective cohort study. Andrologia, e13505.
Attaman, J. A., Toth, T. L., Furtado, J., Campos, H., Hauser, R., & Chavarro, J. E. (2012). Dietary fat and semen quality among men attending a fertility clinic. Human reproduction, 27(5), 1466-1474.
Jensen, T. K., Heitmann, B. L., Jensen, M. B., Halldorsson, T. I., Andersson, A. M., Skakkebæk, N. E.,...& Lassen, T. H. (2013). High dietary intake of saturated fat is associated with reduced semen quality among 701 young Danish men from the general population. The American journal of clinical nutrition, 97(2), 411-418.

109 Jensen, T. K., Heitmann, B. L., Jensen, M. B., Halldorsson, T. I., Andersson, A. M., Skakkebæk, N. E.,...& Lassen, T. H. (2013). High dietary intake of saturated fat is associated with reduced semen quality among 701 young Danish men from the general population. The American journal of clinical nutrition, 97(2), 411-418.

110 Mendiola, J., Torres-Cantero, A. M., Moreno-Grau, J. M., Ten, J., Roca, M., Moreno-Grau, S., & Bernabeu, R. (2009). Food intake and its relationship with semen quality: a case-control study. Fertility and sterility, 91(3), 812-818.

111 Ricci, E., Noli, S., Ferrari, S., La Vecchia, I., Castiglioni, M., Cipriani, S.,...& Agostoni, C. (2020). Fatty acids, food groups and semen variables in men referring to an Italian Fertility Clinic: Cross-sectional analysis of a prospective cohort study. Andrologia, e13505.

112 Salas-Huetos, A., Babio, N., Carrell, D. T., Bulló, M., & Salas-Salvadó, J. (2019). Adherence to the Mediterranean diet is positively associated with sperm motility: A cross-sectional analysis. Scientific reports, 9(1), 1-8.

113 González, F., Considine, R. V., Abdelhadi, O. A., & Acton, A. J. (2019). Saturated fat ingestion promotes lipopolysaccharide-mediated inflammation and insulin resistance in polycystic ovary syndrome. The Journal of Clinical Endocrinology & Metabolism, 104(3), 934-946.

114 González, F., Considine, R. V., Abdelhadi, O. A., & Acton, A. J. (2020). Inflammation triggered by saturated fat ingestion is linked to insulin resistance and hyperandrogenism in polycystic ovary syndrome. The Journal of Clinical Endocrinology & Metabolism, 105(6), dgaa108.

115 González, F., Considine, R. V., Abdelhadi, O. A., & Acton, A. J. (2020). Inflammation triggered by saturated fat ingestion is linked to insulin resistance and hyperandrogenism in polycystic ovary syndrome. The Journal of Clinical Endocrinology & Metabolism, 105(6), dgaa108.
Gonzalez, F., Considine, R. V., Abdelhadi, O. A., & Acton, A. J. (2016). Anti-inflammatory therapy suppresses proinflammatory cytokine secretion from mononuclear cells and reduces hyperandrogenism in lean women with polycystic ovary syndrome (PCOS). Fertility and Sterility, 106(3), e32.

116 Yang, K., Zeng, L., Bao, T., & Ge, J. (2018). Effectiveness of Omega-3 fatty acid for polycystic ovary syndrome: A systematic review and meta-analysis. Reproductive Biology and Endocrinology, 16(1), 27.

Jamilian M, Samimi M, Mirhosseini N, Afshar Ebrahimi F, Aghadavod E, Talaee R, et al. The influences of vitamin D and omega-3 co-supplementation on clinical, metabolic and genetic parameters in women with polycystic ovary syndrome. J Affect Disord. 2018;238:32–38

Rahmani, E., Samimi, M., Ebrahimi, F. A., Foroozanfard, F., Ahmadi, S., Rahimi, M.,...& Memarzadeh, M. R. (2017). The effects of omega-3 fatty acids and vitamin E co-supplementation on gene expression of lipoprotein (a) and oxidized low-density lipoprotein, lipid profiles and biomarkers of oxidative stress in patients with polycystic ovary syndrome. Molecular and cellular endocrinology, 439, 247-255.

Made in the USA
Monee, IL
17 February 2023

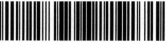

28012166R00122